Calculating X-ray Tube Spectra

Series in Medical Physics and Biomedical Engineering
Series Editors: Kwan Hoong Ng, E. Russell Ritenour, Slavik Tabakov,

Recent books in the series:

Calculating X-ray Tube Spectra

Analytical and Monte Carlo Approaches

Gavin Poludniowski
Artur Omar
Pedro Andreo

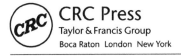

CRC Press
Taylor & Francis Group
Boca Raton London New York

CRC Press is an imprint of the
Taylor & Francis Group, an **informa** business

First edition published 2022
by CRC Press
6000 Broken Sound Parkway NW, Suite 300, Boca Raton, FL 33487-2742

and by CRC Press
4 Park Square, Milton Park, Abingdon, Oxon, OX14 4RN

CRC Press is an imprint of Taylor & Francis Group, LLC

ISBN: 978-0-367-52084-7 (hbk)
ISBN: 978-0-367-52491-3 (pbk)
ISBN: 978-1-003-05816-8 (ebk)

DOI: 10.1201/9781003058168

Publisher's note: This book has been prepared from camera-ready copy provided by the authors

Contents

Preface

The authors of this book have, for many years, been involved in modelling x-ray tubes and using the predictions of the models in practical applications. This monograph constitutes a distillation of our knowledge and experience. We hope it will be of theoretical interest and practical use to scientists working with x-ray tubes, whether in routine or research settings.

The first chapter of this book gives an outline of the book structure and coverage and we refer the reader there for greater specifics. However, we will highlight here that this book covers both analytical models (theoretical, empirical, or semi-empirical) and simulation using the Monte Carlo method. We feel that a comprehensive treatment of the topic of modelling x-ray tubes, which we attempt here, requires consideration of both approaches. It is also our hope that this book can provide a (relatively) easy introduction for those intending to begin working with Monte Carlo simulations.

The history of modelling x-ray tube is long (over 100 years) and we have included a considerable amount of historical material. We hope the reader will indulge our interest in the "archaeology" of x-ray tube models, as the seeds of many modern approaches can be seen in the pioneering early work.

As well as background material and modelling, the book covers practical applications using freely available spectrum modelling software. In these applications, we show how the predictions of x-ray models can be used for predicting beam quality, dosimetry, and image quality optimization.

Any writing project requires a huge investment in time from the authors, including many hours away from family and friends. So we thank our families for their patience and support and belief in the value of this book. We hope that you, the reader, will find value in it too.

Gavin Poludniowski
Artur Omar
Pedro Andreo

1st November 2021
Stockholm, Sweden

Author affiliations

Gavin Poludniowski, PhD

Medical Radiation Physics & Nuclear Medicine
Karolinska University Hospital, Stockholm, Sweden

Department of Clinical Science, Intervention & Technology (CLINTEC)
Karolinska Institutet, Stockholm, Sweden

Artur Omar, PhD

Medical Radiation Physics & Nuclear Medicine
Karolinska University Hospital, Stockholm, Sweden

Department of Oncology-Pathology (ONKPAT)
Karolinska Institutet, Stockholm, Sweden

Prof. Pedro Andreo

Department of Oncology-Pathology (ONKPAT)
Karolinska Institutet, Stockholm, Sweden

Medical Radiation Physics & Nuclear Medicine
Karolinska University Hospital, Stockholm, Sweden

CHAPTER 1

Introduction

T HIS book is concerned with calculating the x-ray spectra emitted from x-ray tubes. This chapter sets out why and how we do this, the topics of the book and highlights software that can be used as supporting tools.

1.1   WHY WE CALCULATE X-RAY SPECTRA

X-ray tubes are used in a variety of fields, including medical imaging, low- and medium energy x-ray radiotherapy, material science, and industrial testing. The optimal characteristics of an x-ray beam can vary widely from application to application and hence x-ray tube design does also. Even for a given x-ray tube, there are adjustable parameters such as the tube potential, exposure setting, and filtration that considerably affect the properties of the beam.

While experimental determination of beam characteristics such as *half-value layer* and *air kerma* are possible (and often important), it is not feasible to make exhaustive measurements of every combination of tube parameter selection. Further some metrics, such as the *x-ray fluence* for a beam, are not practical to determine experimentally in most settings. This is where spectrum models can be invaluable.

1.2   HOW WE CALCULATE X-RAY SPECTRA

The sophistication required in modelling an x-ray spectrum is determined by the particular task. A medical physicist working in a hospital might simply want to know how the *half-value layer* of an x-ray beam changes when a filter of known thickness is added to an x-ray tube. There is therefore a need for simple modelling software that can provide predictions of such metrics in a rapid and convenient manner.

DOI: 10.1201/9781003058168-1

A scientist investigating x-ray tube design or performance might use comprehensive *Monte Carlo* software to simulate a tube. This application would include a geometry package capable of representing the x-ray target, tube housing and beam filters, and a detailed and accurate model for the physics of radiation transport, including the scattered radiation. The software might also be capable of simulating the trajectories of electrons in electromagnetic fields as they strike the target. Such complex software exists, is even freely available in some cases, but requires considerable expertise and cannot yield answers immediately.

1.3   COVERAGE AND STRUCTURE OF THIS BOOK

This book is primarily concerned with the x-ray tubes used in diagnostic and interventional radiology, as well as low- and medium-energy radiotherapy. The x-ray tubes considered will be *thick-target* tubes operated in a *reflection* rather than *transmission* geometry. The material for the target anode will be tungsten—or possibly molybdenum in mammography applications—and the range of tube potentials will be from a few kilovolts to several hundred kilovolts. Although this coverage does not address all applications, it covers the most important varieties of x-ray tubes used in medical x-ray imaging and radiotherapy, as well as many other fields.

The approaches discussed will range from analytic models of varying sophistication (theoretical, empirical, and semi-empirical), to modelling with Monte Carlo packages. The emphasis, however, will always be on modelling the spectrum emerging from the tube, rather than accurately modelling the full design of these complex pieces of engineering.

The book is split into three sections: *Background*, *Modelling*, and *Applications*. Each chapter of the *Background* and *Modelling* sections builds on the previous ones. The three chapters in the *Applications* section, however, are entirely independent and can be read in any order.

1.4   ACCOMPANYING SOFTWARE

The reader is likely to get more out of this book if he or she explores the concepts and examples further using some variety of software for predicting x-ray spectra. We will frequently make use of the SpekPy toolkit [1, 2] to produce simple metrics, plots and to provide pedagogic examples. SpekPy is a toolkit for modelling x-ray tube spectra in the Python programming language. It can be used to calculate on- and off-axis spectra for tungsten, molybdenum, and rhodium anodes. The toolkit is distributed free-of-charge under the open-source MIT license.

Although the book content is tailored towards SpekPy and the Python programming language, the reader has other options for exploring x-ray spectra. For example, alternatives in the MATLAB® (MathWorks Inc.,

Natwick, WY, USA) environment exist, as do stand-alone applications. The reader can refer to Chapter 5 for some potential alternatives to SpekPy.

Python scripts to support learning from this book are available in an online repository, at: https://bitbucket.org/caxtus. At the end of each chapter you will find a box like this, informing you of how you can explore the material further with Python and SpekPy. For this chapter, there is a script called *spekpy_demo.py*. This script demonstrates how to use the SpekPy toolkit to generate and plot an x-ray spectrum and how to calculate half-value layers, air kerma and fluence. Make sure you install SpekPy-v2 (version 2) before trying to run it. See: https://bitbucket.org/spekpy/spekpy_release.

I

Background

CHAPTER 2

Basics of x-ray tubes

I N this chapter, we look at some basic features of x-ray tube design and define those aspects important for the modelling approaches presented later in the book.

2.1 EVOLUTION OF THE X-RAY TUBE

When Roentgen discovered x rays in 1895, the technology he used to generate them looked very different from that used today [3]. Roentgen used what is known as a Crookes tube, consisting of a partially evacuated glass bulb. The lack of high vacuum was in fact essential to the operation of this kind of tube, as it relied on a *cold cathode*. The Crookes tube had an anode and cathode and a high potential difference between them—a few kilovolts or more. A complex cascade of ionization processes was initiated under the high potential difference, resulting in positive ions from the residual gas bombarding the cathode and liberating a large number of electrons. The free electrons were then repelled from the cathode and accelerated through the potential difference. Roentgen used a flat aluminium cathode and the resulting stream of electrons struck the wall of the tube enclosure. It was here, in the glass, that x-rays were generated.

After those first historic observations by Roentgen, x-ray tube design evolved rapidly. Gas tubes tailored towards x-ray applications quickly arrived, using *targets* for x-ray production, typically made of metal and also acting as the anode. The second decade of the twentieth century saw a number of innovations that are still relevant today [3]. In 1913, Coolidge introduced the high-vacuum hot-cathode tube that is named after him, allowing greater stability and reliability. A hot cathode means that the electrons providing the tube current were liberated by thermionic emission (from a tungsten filament), rather than ion bombardment. Two years later, Coolidge described the first rotating anode tube, enabling superior heat dissipation. Progress did not stop there. Some other notable developments made over the last 125 years are [4–7]:

DOI: 10.1201/9781003058168-2

- High atomic number targets to increase x-ray production efficiency

- A thick target, often embedded in another metal such as molybdenum or copper, because of their heat dissipation properties

- Tungsten (or tungsten-alloy[1]) is a preferred target material due to its high melting point, strength, and relatively low evaporation under the harsh conditions inside an x-ray tube

- Use of the reflection geometry to provide a useful beam (rather than relying on transmission through the target)

- Innovations in cathode design such as concave cathodes to assist in focusing the electrons onto a focal spot or flat sheet emitters to help control focal-spot size at high tube currents

- Electron traps to capture electrons backscattered from the target surface and reduce extra-focal radiation

- Three-phase or constant potential generators to maintain a more constant tube potential during a radiation exposure

- Ceramic and metal tube casings, with several advantages including increased durability and heat capacity

- Liquid metal bearings to reduce friction and wear and further increase heat dissipation

It is important to realize that x-ray tube development has not followed a straight line, converging towards a single optimal design. Today, there is a huge range of tube types developed for different applications, or even for the same application. The tube of primary interest in this book is a high-vacuum tube with a hot cathode, a thick metal anode acting as the target, and a reflection geometry (see fig. 2.1). The engineering details are mostly inessential for the purposes of this book. However, it is useful to know a few further facts and some basics of terminology.

2.2   X-RAY TUBE ESSENTIALS

2.2.1   X-ray exposure factors

An x-ray exposure can be specified in terms of:

- The tube potential, V, specified in kilovolts (kV)

- The tube current, I, specified in milliamperes (mA)

---

[1] A typical "tungsten" target in fact contains a small percentage of rhenium. As rhenium is adjacent to tungsten in the periodic table and the alloys have a similar density to pure tungsten, this fact is often ignored in modelling, as it will be throughout this book.

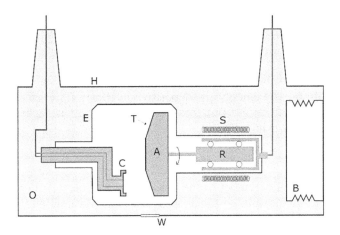

Figure 2.1: Schematic of typical x-ray tube operating in the reflection geometry. A—Anode, B—Expansion bellows (provides space for oil to expand), C—Cathode and heating coil, E—Tube envelope (evacuated), H—Tube housing, O—Cooling dielectric oil, R—Rotor, S—Induction stator, T—Anode target, W—Tube window (aluminium or beryllium). Adapted from wikipedia:User:ChumpusRex, CC BY-SA 3.0 (http://creativecommons.org/licenses/by-sa/3.0), via Wikimedia Commons [8].

- The exposure duration, T, specified in seconds (s)

The tube potential determines the kinetic energy of the electrons striking the target and hence the maximum energy of x rays. The potential is applied by the x-ray generator, which converts AC mains power to a high-voltage DC output [5]. Historically, the waveform of the output potential was far from constant during exposure. The degree of *voltage ripple* in a waveform is defined as the difference between the maximum (peak) and minimum voltage, divided by the maximum voltage [9]. In modern generators, the ripple is typically low, and throughout this book, we will assume a constant potential (i.e., 0% ripple). For some generators, particularly for portable or mobile x-ray units, the ripple may be significant and the tube potential may need to be replaced by an effective value. If the waveform is known, the *practical peak voltage* can be calculated [9–11] or spectral-averaging over the waveform performed [12].

The tube current specifies the charge reaching the target per unit time. The exposure duration specifies the period in which the x-ray tube emits x rays. The number of electrons striking the target, $\mathcal{N}$, is proportional to the tube current and exposure duration product (the mAs):

$$\mathcal{N} = 10^{-3}\frac{IT}{e}, \tag{2.1}$$

where e is the electron charge (1.602×10^{-19} C). The conversion between IT (mAs) and the number of electrons is worth emphasizing as some results for x-ray production presented in this book are expressed per mAs and others per incident electron.

The energy, W, deposited in a target during exposure is,

$$W = VIT, \tag{2.2}$$

assuming that the tube potential is constant during exposure.

Nearly all of the energy is deposited as heat. The efficiency of x-ray production (the proportion of energy emitted as x rays) follows the approximate relationship [13],

$$\epsilon = 10^{-6}ZV, \tag{2.3}$$

where Z is the atomic number of the target. The efficiency is therefore low, at around 1% in the kilovoltage range, even for a high atomic number material like tungsten. This has meant that heat dissipation has been a constant consideration in x-ray tube design, to ensure the desired power output is obtained without melting or otherwise destroying the target.

2.2.2 The x-ray spectrum and filtration

The x-ray spectrum is the distribution of x rays over x-ray energy (see Section 4.1.1). An important question to consider is *where* the spectrum is specified. The spectrum emitted within the target is never identical to that exiting the tube or reaching a detector.

X rays are produced at varying depths within the target, through both bremsstrahlung and atomic relaxation processes (see Chapter 3). A proportion of these x rays are attenuated before they escape. This is referred to as *self-filtration* by the target.

Everything else the beam must pass through before exiting the tube housing is referred to as *inherent filtration*. This includes the tube exit window, possibly a layer of oil between the tube and the tube housing and the housing itself. The tube exit window is often made of a layer of beryllium, which is highly radiation transparent. The window is typically 1 mm or thicker, to withstand atmospheric pressure against the vacuum. In applications where the low-energy x-rays (below about 15 keV) are not useful, a material such as aluminium can be used instead.

In addition, extra filtration, often aluminium or copper, may be added to modify the beam. The purpose is to remove low-energy x rays too *soft* to be useful and to tune the penetrative capabilities of the beam to the particular task. Such filtration is referred to as *added filtration*. Most commonly this is used to *harden* the beam, with lower energy x rays being preferentially removed. This is not always the case, however, as the K-edge of some materials may be taken of advantage for the increased suppression of x rays of energy above the K-edge. In such a situation, the material acts more as a band-pass filter.

Additional functional components such as a reflecting mirror for a light field or a monitor ionization chamber may be present in the beam. These typically are very minor contributions to attenuation of the beam but can be classified as inherent or added filtration. Air is also present between the x-ray tube and the detector. For low tube potentials (below about 100 kV) with minimal added filtration, the effect of air attenuation and scattering on the x-ray fluence may be significant.

Section 4.2 provides more in-depth detail on specifying the penetrative characteristics of beams, otherwise referred to as the *beam quality*.

2.2.3 The line-focus principle and the heel effect

The region on the target that the incident electrons are focused upon is called the *focal spot*. The focal-spot size limits the spatial resolution of x-ray images, although geometrical magnification also plays a role. In 1918, a surgeon named Goetze proposed the *line-focus principle* [14]. This is illustrated in fig. 2.2. The insight was that in a reflection geometry as depicted, the effective focal-spot size as observed in the beam's-eye-view is dependent on the angle of the anode. Goetze suggested using a rectangular focal spot stretched considerably in one direction, combined with a shallow anode angle. The area in which the heat was deposited could therefore be made larger while still maintaining the same effective focal-spot size from the patient's perspective.

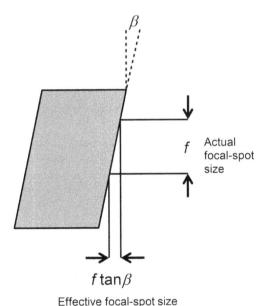

Figure 2.2: An illustration of the line-focus principle for a reflection mode x-ray tube. The focal-spot size is determined by the width of the incident electron beam (horizontal, right-to-left). The effective focal-spot size of the resulting x rays (vertical, top-to-bottom) is reduced by a factor $\tan \beta$.

The drawback to employing a shallow anode angle is that it limits the useful angles of emission for an x-ray beam. There is a limit for the width of the beam defined by the grazing angle with the anode surface. In addition, because the x rays are emitted at depth in the target, as the emission angle approaches the limit the x rays must pass through an increased thickness of target material to escape. This reduces the fluence. The phenomenon is known as the *anode heel effect*. This is illustrated in fig. 2.3 for a tube potential of 80 kV and a total filtration of 2.5 mm of aluminium. The fluence (per mAs) at a plane 100 cm from the focus is plotted against the position, for anode angles of 12° and 24°. The usable beam width is less for the lower anode angle. This comes, however, with a factor of 2 reduction in effective focal spot size $(\tan 12° / \tan 24° \approx 2)$.

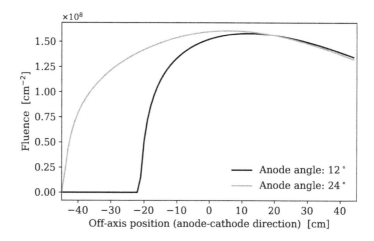

Figure 2.3: An illustration of the anode heel effect for anode angles of 12° and 24°. The magnitude of the heel effect was calculated using the SpekPy toolkit for: 80 kV tube potential, 2.5 mm Al filtration, 1 mAs tube current, and 100 cm source-to-detector distance.

2.3   UNDERSTANDING X-RAY TUBE DESIGN

Understanding the demands of a particular application helps in understanding the x-ray tube design. This is of importance to x-ray beam modelling, since design factors, particularly the anode angle, target material, and filter materials will affect the beam characteristics. The emphasis here will primarily be on medical field, but the applications within this broad area have varying requirements and similarities to many other fields.

In medical x-ray imaging, low noise images must be obtained in the image receptor after the beam has been attenuated many-fold by the thickness of the patient. The exposure times often need to be short in order to freeze the anatomy in a stationary position. Many images may also need to be acquired in sequence, either to visualize physiological processes or to capture multiple views for tomographic reconstruction. In addition to this, while variable, the demands on spatial resolution are always high, requiring a small effective focal spot (typically 0.1 to 2 mm) [15, 16]. These requirements combine to make high power density demands on an x-ray tube. For this reason, in addition to employing rotating anodes, the line-focus principle is exploited with anode angles that are shallow and typically in the range 7° to 15° [15].

In Computed Tomography (CT), the power demands on an x-ray tube are particularly high [17]. In a fraction of a second, the x-ray source might rotate around a patient, with the detector capturing hundreds or thousands of image frames. Fortunately, the required width of the beam along the axis of rotation of the source is often relatively short. This enables the anode-cathode direction of the tube to be aligned with the rotation axis and particularly shallow anode angles to be used. In other medical applications, the anode angles are typically somewhat larger, while still employing rotating anodes, but these features are by no means universal. Stationary anodes with larger anode angles (up to around 20°) may be employed where a wide or highly uniform beam is required and the demand is for a relatively low but steady output, or where the detector can be placed close to the source. Such applications can include, in some situations, imaging in surgery using C-arm systems, or dental x-ray [7].

Mammography and imaging of the breast, in general, have some unique demands [16]. The breast can be considered, for most purposes, as purely soft-tissue[2], and the average thickness of compressed breast is just a few cm. High soft-tissue contrast is required to visualize cancerous lesions. This entails a less penetrative x-ray beam and consequently a lower tube potential. Although tungsten is often used as a target in modern digital mammography, other materials such as molybdenum may alternatively be employed to exploit the fact that their characteristic radiation is of suitable energy. Added filtration of molybdenum or rhodium may also be used, exploiting the enhanced absorption above their K-edges to manipulate the quality of the beam. In mammography, as well as soft-tissue contrast, particularly high spatial resolution is also required to detect small high-contrast micro-calcifications. The effective focal-spot size must therefore be small: 0.1 to 0.4 mm [16]. Shallow anode angles may be employed, but the tube tilted to obtain a sufficient field-of-view given the small anode angle. The heel effect may even be exploited and the thinner tip of the breast (requiring less fluence) oriented towards the anode, where increased target self-absorption reduces the number of x rays reaching the patient.

Medical applications of x-ray tubes do not always include imaging and imaging applications are not always medical. The demands on tubes are varied. Stationary target x-ray tubes with large anode angles (20° or larger) are still used for radiotherapy of superficial lesions [18, 19]. In this application

---

[2]Whereas when discussing radiation beam quality, *soft* and *hard* refer to the penetrative properties of the beam, when discussing biological tissues, *soft* refers to non-bony tissue, such as muscle or fat.

a focal spot size of several mm is permissible, the patient's skin can be placed relatively close to the source and the exposure can be spread over many seconds. Stationary anode tubes with large anode angles are also typically used by Primary Standards Dosimetry Laboratories (PSDLs) [20, 21]. It is worth knowing that the reference beam qualities that they provide are usually based on measurements with x-ray tubes quite different from a typical medical x-ray tube. X-ray tubes manufactured for industrial inspection are also usually of stationary anode design but with a range of focal spot sizes (from sub-mm to around 10 mm) and anode angles (from $10°$ to more than $30°$) [22, 23].

In some applications, the typical x-ray tube and its reflection geometry have proved limiting. A good example is Micro-CT, used in many fields for tomographic imaging of relatively small objects with extraordinary spatial resolution. Here, thin transmission targets may be used [24, 25]. To achieve a very high resolution *and* a high power source, radically different technology such as a liquid metal (Metal Jet) target may even be employed [26]. This book, however, focuses exclusively on the technology that is still at the core of most x-ray tubes: a solid thick target.

2.4 REPRESENTATIONS OF TUBES IN MODELS

2.4.1 Simplified analytical models

In 1945, Coolidge and Charlton wrote that [3]:

"Since its birth, the roentgen-ray tube has undergone many radical changes. The general method of producing roentgen rays is, however, still the same, namely by accelerating electrons to a high velocity and then suddenly stopping them by collision with a solid body, the so-called target."

This quote encapsulates the essential facts necessary for modelling the output of an x-ray tube: electrons hit a target and slow down, losing some of that energy by emitting x rays.

Figure 2.4 shows the critical features of x-ray tube design for the purposes of the analytical models discussed in this book. We define an analytical model as any empirical, semi-empirical, or purely theoretical model that does not rely on random sampling methods to produce a prediction of an x-ray spectrum. This is in contrast to simulation methods based on the Monte Carlo transport of electrons and x-rays. The plane depicted in the figure is the canonical one shown in most diagrams in the literature.

In analytical models, the complexity of tube design is typically distilled down to the idea of a stream of electrons hitting a solid block. The size of the focal spot is usually assumed to be zero, since it is the calculation of the x-ray spectrum that is of primary interest rather than spatial resolution. The tilt of the tube (α) and the anode angle (β) are defined with respect to a central axis. The *take-off* angle (φ) is the angle of the x rays with respect to the target surface. This take-off angle determines the degree to which the target attenuates x rays before they escape the tube. This depends on the tilt and

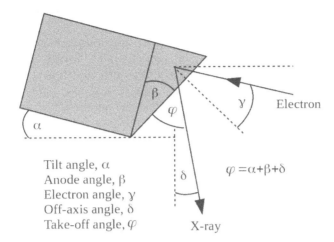

Tilt angle, α
Anode angle, β
Electron angle, γ
Off-axis angle, δ
Take-off angle, φ

$\varphi = \alpha + \beta + \delta$

X-ray

Figure 2.4: The in-plane geometry assumed for analytical models of an x-ray tube.

anode angle and the off-axis angle (δ). The angle of x-ray emissions relative to the central axis, in the direction orthogonal to the depicted plane, is the out-of-plane angle (ϑ).

At first glance, the angle of incidence of the electron beam to the target (γ) may also seem to be important. Often, in books and articles, the electron beam is depicted as travelling at a right angle to the central axis (as in fig. 2.2a). This may or may not be the case, for a given tube, but if it is the case, then the electrons would appear to strike the target at an oblique angle. This is a significant issue for analytical models because many assume that the electrons penetrate into the target in a straight line, continuing at the incident angle [27–30].

However, since the electric field lines in a conductor are always perpendicular to the surface, the trajectory of incident electrons will be modified such that they are deflected towards normal incidence as they approach the target. The true angle of incidence will be somewhere between the oblique angle of approach and zero degrees. Detailed simulations suggest that it may typically be closer to the latter [31]. In any case, the electrons quickly undergo multiple elastic scattering in the target and their direction at depth rapidly loses correlation with the original trajectory.

Although software for calculating x-ray spectra is often used as "black boxes" by users, it is worth understanding their assumptions and limitations. Chapters 5 and 6 provide a review of some major analytical models, including empirical approaches.

Once the x-ray spectrum emerging from the target has been calculated, inherent and added filtration is applied using tabulations of linear attenuation coefficients. Since it is only the primary radiation that is modelled, it is generally assumed that the order and spatial location of filters are irrelevant.

2.4.2 Beyond analytical models

Even the simplified picture described in the previous section is complicated by the complex electron and x-ray interactions in the target (see Chapter 3). Electrons do not penetrate in a straight line into the target, as is assumed in many analytic models, rather they scatter and lose energy in random processes. In fact, with normal incidence to the anode, for a tungsten target and kilovoltage energies, around 50% of the incident electrons backscatter out of the target again [32]. Some will be accelerated back towards the target but hit it away from the focal spot. This is often the major component of so-called *extra-focal* or *off-focal* radiation, which contributes to dose but with little or no contribution to image quality. This extra-focal contribution varies from negligible to substantial but is always much less than the focal component [31]. Although it is possible to approach the problem of extra-focal radiation and a finite spot size using analytical models, a natural approach is to use Monte Carlo simulation packages. Likewise, Monte Carlo is the natural approach to calculating other secondary components to the radiation field such as x-ray scatter from the housing, collimators, and filters.

In Monte Carlo simulation, in addition to specifying spot sizes, the geometry of the tube must be defined. Figure 2.5 depicts a simplified representation of an x-ray tube displayed in the Graphical User Interface (GUI) of the BEAMnrc Monte Carlo user code [33]. The model is crude but includes the most salient components: a thick angled tungsten target, a slab of beryllium representing an exit window and lead collimation that limits the beam. A column of air has also been placed between the tube and the measurement point, where the number and energies of x rays are to be scored. The sophistication of the geometric model will depend on the task, accuracy required and the detail of tube specifications available from the manufacturer. A tube representation may be as simple as that illustrated or include a finely detailed geometry based on tube schematics. It may also, if the simulation code incorporates the functionality, allow the simulation of the transport of the electrons in the electric field [34,35]. Crucially, if the user wants to accurately model scatter and beam penumbra, any components such as collimators and filtration must be correctly positioned with the correct compositions allocated.

In many Monte Carlo simulation programs, a variety of physics models, algorithms, and transport thresholds can be selected. This may be because the most accurate model is unknown, or varies between simulation scenarios. Or it may simply be that the time required for the simulation can be reduced in some circumstances, with suitable selections, without loss of accuracy. Regardless, such choices can affect predictions and appropriate selections should be made. This can be daunting for the novice. Chapter 7 provides further discussion of Monte Carlo codes and some of the issues to consider.

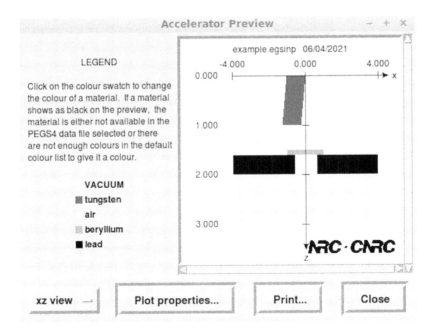

Figure 2.5: An example representation of an x-ray tube in the BEAMnrc user code of the EGSnrc Monte Carlo code system [33]. The target is inclined at a 14° angle and the electron beam is incident along the x-axis (right-to-left).

The Python script used to generate fig. 2.3 is available in the book's online software repository, at: https://bitbucket.org/caxtus. The script is called *heel_effect.py* and uses the SpekPy-v2 toolkit. Try changing the beam filtration in the script and running it. In the region where both beams are non-zero, do the beam profiles become more or less similar as the filtration is increased? Can you explain this?

CHAPTER 3

X-ray production

T HIS chapter provides an introduction to the physics of x-ray production in an x-ray tube anode, including the transport of electrons, and the particle-atom interactions that generate x rays.

3.1 ELECTRON TRANSPORT

As discussed in Chapter 2, conventional x-ray tubes include a conducting anode that is irradiated by electrons released by thermionic emission from a heated metallic wire coil that acts as a cathode. The released electrons are accelerated by an electric field in the vacuum space between the anode and cathode and enter the anode normally, or near normally, according to finite element simulations [36]; recall that electric field lines are perpendicular to the surface of a conductor. As the electrons penetrate into the anode, they lose kinetic energy in Coulomb interactions with target atoms. Most of the incident kinetic energy is eventually converted into heat, with only a small fraction of the energy (typically less than one percent) lost through the emission of electromagnetic radiation, that is, bremsstrahlung and characteristic x rays.

Different interaction processes produce x rays, as outlined in fig. 3.1 and further described in Sections 3.2 and 3.3. These interactions occur as a result of the electron-photon cascade process initiated by incident electrons penetrating the anode (i.e., target). Therefore, before delving into how x rays are produced, let us consider the main features of the electron penetration into a thick target, as it defines the x-ray radiation emanating from an x-ray tube.

Electrons penetrating an x-ray target undergo multiple elastic scatterings and eventually lose all of their kinetic energy in inelastic collisions and radiative emissions in the electric field of target atoms. The combination of multiple scattering and energy loss causes the electrons to attain a broader energy spectrum (fig. 3.3) and angular distribution (fig. 3.4) with penetration depth. It should be noted that for an isotropic medium with randomly oriented atoms, the angular distribution of the penetrating electrons is axially

DOI: 10.1201/9781003058168-3

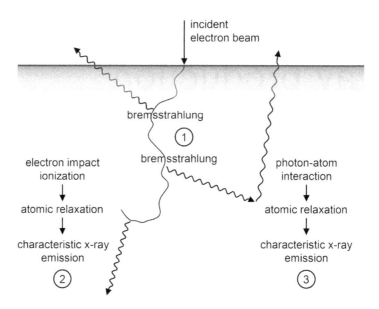

Figure 3.1: Electrons penetrating a target produce x rays as a result of the following processes: (1) an electron that is scattered in the electric field generated by atomic electrons and nuclei emits bremsstrahlung with energy equal to the electron kinetic energy loss; (2) an electron knocks out an inner-shell electron, and the resulting ion relaxes by emitting an x ray with characteristic energy; (3) a bremsstrahlung photon ionizes a target atom by photoelectric absorption or Compton scattering, and the resulting ion relaxes by emitting an x ray with characteristic energy.

symmetric, which means that it can be fully characterized by the polar angle about the incident direction.

The effects of multiple scattering and energy loss can be observed in the electron number depth distribution (electron fluence integrated over the lateral plane), shown in fig. 3.2. At first, the number of electrons builds up due to the injection of secondary (knock-on) electrons generated in inelastic collisions, and due to multiple elastic scatterings broadening the angular distribution and making electrons pass through a given depth more than once. Some electrons are backscattered and ejected from the target, thus reducing the x-ray yield. After the initial build-up, the number of electrons is reduced as they are slowed down to rest by repeated kinetic energy losses. The penetration depth is not deeper than about half the continuous-slowing-down-approximation (CSDA) range (see eq. (4.12)), due to multiple scattering causing the electrons to take a rather tortuous path in the target rather than following a straight line.

The electron angular distribution (see fig. 3.4) is initially strongly correlated with the incident direction, but as the mean energy decreases, scattering becomes increasingly important and the electron angular distribution

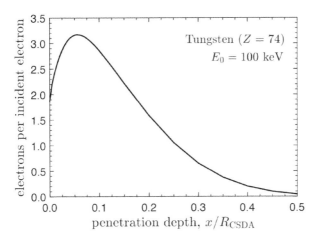

Figure 3.2: Electron number (electron fluence integrated over the lateral plane) at depth in tungsten for 100 keV incident electrons. The results were obtained using the PENELOPE Monte Carlo system [35] with the electron transport cut-off energy set to 5 keV.

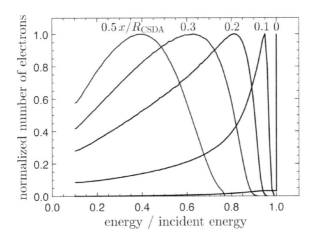

Figure 3.3: Electron energy spectra in tungsten for 100 keV incident electrons. The distributions correspond to the indicated penetration depths scaled by the CSDA range (x/R_{CSDA}), and they are normalized to their respective maximum. The results were obtained using the PENELOPE Monte Carlo system [35] with the electron transport cut-off energy set to 5 keV.

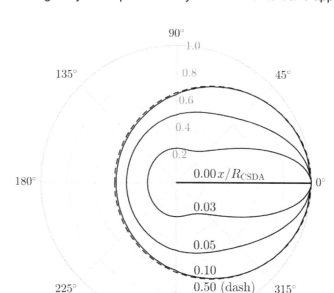

Figure 3.4: Electron angular distributions in tungsten for 100 keV incident electrons. The distributions correspond to the indicated penetration depths scaled by the CSDA range (x/R_{CSDA}), and they are normalized to their respective maximum. The results were obtained using the PENELOPE Monte Carlo system [35] with the electron transport cut-off energy set to 5 keV.

broadens. After sufficient scattering, the direction of motion becomes so diffuse that the angular distribution becomes very broad, albeit with more electrons forward scattered (polar angle between 0 and 90°) than backscattered. In this region, which is sometimes referred to as the region of *diffusion*, the angular distribution no longer changes with increasing penetration depth. The region of diffusion begins at a depth of about 0.1 times the CSDA range for typical incident electron energies.

As the electrons penetrate the target, they undergo various interaction processes, some of which result in radiative emissions. These emissions occur either in Coulomb interactions with target atoms (bremsstrahlung) or by fluorescence following atomic ionization by electron impact or photon interactions (characteristic x-ray emission). The fundamentals of these processes are outlined in the following Sections 3.2 and 3.3.

3.2 BREMSSTRAHLUNG PRODUCTION

Consider an electron with kinetic energy E traveling in direction $\hat{\boldsymbol{\Omega}}_e$ in the electric field generated by atomic electrons and nuclei. The electron may emit a bremsstrahlung photon with energy k in direction $\hat{\boldsymbol{\Omega}}_\gamma$ when scattered by the Coulomb field. For an isotropic medium with randomly oriented atoms, the intrinsic angular distribution of the bremsstrahlung emission can be treated as axially symmetric and the photon emission direction can as such be expressed in terms of the polar angle, $\cos\theta = \hat{\boldsymbol{\Omega}}_e \cdot \hat{\boldsymbol{\Omega}}_\gamma$. For a complete treatment of bremsstrahlung emission, the direction of the scattered electron also has to be considered. However, in condensed matter, the angular deflection of the electron following bremsstrahlung emission can usually be neglected, as it is obscured by the several orders of magnitude more frequently occurring elastic scatterings.

Ignoring polarization effects[1]—which is to assume a summation over final (spin and photon) polarizations and an average over initial polarizations—the bremsstrahlung process in a target material with an atomic number Z can be fully described by an atomic cross section double differential in photon energy and photon emission direction,

$$\frac{\mathrm{d}^2\sigma_{\mathrm{br}}(k, \hat{\boldsymbol{\Omega}}_e \cdot \hat{\boldsymbol{\Omega}}_\gamma; Z, E)}{\mathrm{d}k\,\mathrm{d}\hat{\boldsymbol{\Omega}}_\gamma} = \frac{Z^2}{\beta_i^2}\frac{1}{k}\chi(k; Z, E)\,S(\hat{\boldsymbol{\Omega}}_e \cdot \hat{\boldsymbol{\Omega}}_\gamma; k, Z, E), \quad (3.1)$$

where β_i is the initial electron velocity in units of the speed of light in vacuum, χ is the scaled energy-weighted bremsstrahlung cross section differential in photon energy k, and S is the shape function of the bremsstrahlung angular distribution. The right-hand side of the above equation is a convenient factorization of the double differential cross section [39], as it allows for the photon energy and the photon emission angle to be determined separately and efficiently in numerical calculations. This factorization is therefore typically employed in Monte Carlo transport codes.

The scaled energy-weighted bremsstrahlung cross section and the shape function can be expressed, respectively, as,

$$\chi(k; Z, E) = \frac{\beta_i^2}{Z^2}k\frac{\mathrm{d}\sigma_{\mathrm{br}}(k; Z, E)}{\mathrm{d}k}, \quad (3.2)$$

and

$$S(\hat{\boldsymbol{\Omega}}_e \cdot \hat{\boldsymbol{\Omega}}_\gamma; k, Z, E) = \frac{\mathrm{d}^2\sigma_{\mathrm{br}}}{\mathrm{d}k\,\mathrm{d}\hat{\boldsymbol{\Omega}}_\gamma}\left(\frac{\mathrm{d}\sigma_{\mathrm{br}}}{\mathrm{d}k}\right)^{-1}. \quad (3.3)$$

Numerical results for these functions, obtained by calculations in partial-wave expansions [39, 40], are presented in figs. 3.5 and 3.6. Notice that χ varies relatively slowly with E and k/E for a given element Z due to the use of the scaling factor $(\beta_i/Z)^2 k$.

---

[1]Bremsstrahlung emissions do exhibit polarization, even for an unpolarized electron beam. This has measurable effects, such as introducing dependence on the azimuthal as well as polar angle into the angular distribution of Compton scattering. The degree of polarization depends on electron energy, x-ray emission energy, target atomic number, and emission angle in a rather complicated manner [37,38]. It is relatively weak for thick targets, however, and is not considered explicitly in this book (i.e. polarization states are summed).

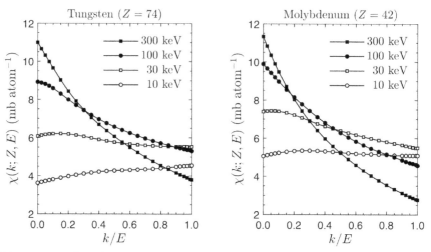

Figure 3.5: Scaled energy-weighted bremsstrahlung cross section (eq. (3.1)) as a function of the photon energy scaled by the initial electron energy, k/E. The values have been extracted from the PENELOPE materials database [35] (based on partial-wave expansions [39]), and correspond to the indicated initial electron energies.

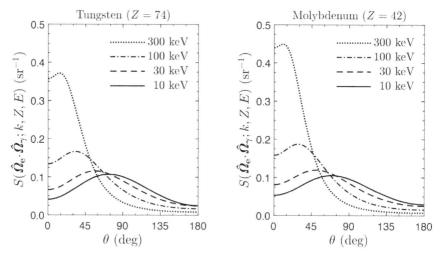

Figure 3.6: Intrinsic bremsstrahlung angular distribution (eq. (3.2)) for photons emitted with half of the initial electron energy, $k/E = 0.5$. The values have been extracted from PENELOPE materials database [35] (based on partial-wave expansions [39]), and correspond to the indicated initial electron energies.

A considerable body of theory on the bremsstrahlung cross section has been developed over the years. In 1959, Koch and Motz [13] published a comprehensive review in which they outlined various analytical theories for the single differential (photon energy), double differential (photon energy and emission angle), and triple differential (photon energy, and photon and electron emission angle) cross section. The analytical formulas included in their review were based on the first Born approximation with the electron states represented by plane waves (PWBA theory). They also presented a set of analytical and empirical correction factors that account for Coulomb effects not included in the Born approximation, as well as the screening of the central potential (the nucleus) by atomic electrons.

More recent advances were summarized in the review by Pratt *et al.* [41], which includes relativistic partial-wave calculations that overcome the inherent limitation of PWBA in that higher-order Coulomb distortion effects are accounted for. The omission of higher order terms in the electron wave function assumes that the distortion of the plane waves by the Coulomb field of the nucleus is very weak, a description that does not hold for high-Z materials and low-energy electrons [42].

Commonly used cross sections for the intrinsic bremsstrahlung energy and angular distribution are described in the following Sections 3.2.1 and 3.2.2.

3.2.1 Intrinsic energy distribution

The bremsstrahlung cross section differential in energy has been calculated by Seltzer and Berger [40, 43] at the National Institute of Standards and Technology. Their results have been implemented in most contemporary Monte Carlo transport codes, and they have also been adopted in ICRU Report 90 [44] for the radiative energy-loss cross section. Seltzer and Berger calculated the bremsstrahlung cross section for electrons as the sum of two terms,

$$\frac{\mathrm{d}\sigma_{\mathrm{br}}}{\mathrm{d}k} = \frac{\mathrm{d}\sigma_{\mathrm{br}}^{\mathrm{n}}}{\mathrm{d}k} + Z\frac{\mathrm{d}\sigma_{\mathrm{br}}^{\mathrm{e}}}{\mathrm{d}k}, \tag{3.4}$$

where $\mathrm{d}\sigma_{\mathrm{br}}^{\mathrm{n}}/\mathrm{d}k$ is the cross section for bremsstrahlung produced in the field of the screened atomic nucleus, and $Z(\mathrm{d}\sigma_{\mathrm{br}}^{\mathrm{e}}/\mathrm{d}k)$ represents bremsstrahlung produced in the field of Z atomic electrons.

The electron-nucleus bremsstrahlung cross section was calculated by combining different theories based on the initial electron kinetic energy:

- For 1 keV $\leq E \leq 2$ MeV, the results are from numerical partial-wave calculations by Pratt *et al.* [45] for the emission of bremsstrahlung in the electric field generated by a static screened Coulomb potential. Their calculations are considered to be some of the most reliable results available for the electron-nucleus bremsstrahlung in this energy range, with the relative uncertainty estimated to be no more than 10%. It is worth emphasizing that the partial-wave results cover the full range of energies considered in this book.

- For $50 \text{ MeV} \leq E \leq 10 \text{ GeV}$, the cross section was evaluated by combining results from the high-energy theory of Davies, Bethe, Maximon, and Olsen (DBMO),

$$\frac{d\sigma_{br}^n}{dk} = \left(\frac{d\sigma_{br}^n}{dk}\right)_{3BN} + \delta_{screen} + \delta_{Coul}, \tag{3.5}$$

where $(d\sigma_{br}^n/dk)_{3BN}$ is the PWBA cross section by Bethe and Heitler [46] for a non-screened Coulomb potential (formula 3BN in ref. [13]), with δ_{screen} correcting for screening effects based on high-energy approximations (formula 3BSb in ref. [13]), and δ_{Coul} being an additive Coulomb correction that accounts for the distortion of the plane wave by the Coulomb field of the nucleus. The relative standard uncertainty was for this set of cross sections estimated to be 3–5%.

- For $2 \text{ MeV} < E < 50 \text{ MeV}$, a numerical least-squares cubic-spline interpolation scheme was used to combine the low-energy results obtained by partial-wave calculations and the high-energy results calculated according to eq. (3.5). The relative standard uncertainty was for this energy range estimated to be 5–10%.

The electron-electron bremsstrahlung cross section was calculated in the following form,

$$\frac{d\sigma_{br}^e}{dk} = f_{e\text{-}e}\left(\frac{d\sigma_{br}^e}{dk}\right)_H + \delta_{screen}^e, \tag{3.6}$$

where $(d\sigma_{br}^e/dk)_H$ is the Born-approximation formula by Haug [47] for an unscreened free electron, including recoil effects; δ_{screen}^e is a correction for the screening of the field of the atomic electrons based on Wheeler and Lamb's high-energy theory [48], which also takes into account atomic binding; and $f_{e\text{-}e}$ is a multiplicative Coulomb correction [49].

Tessier and Kawrakow [50] have recently calculated electron-electron bremsstrahlung cross sections for the EGSnrc Monte Carlo system [34] (referred to as the NRC cross sections) that explicitly account for the effects of atomic binding. Note, however, that the electron-electron bremsstrahlung contribution is minimal for medium- and high-Z targets. Recall that the production of bremsstrahlung in the field of atomic electrons is proportional to Z (because each electron acts as a separate scattering centre), whereas the production of bremsstrahlung in the field of the nucleus is proportional to Z^2 (because it is related to the square of the interaction strength, which is itself proportional to the number of nuclear protons).

3.2.2 Intrinsic angular distribution

This section provides an introduction to the various theories for the intrinsic bremsstrahlung angular distribution, i.e., the shape function, developed over the years, with a more comprehensive analysis available in ref. [51].

Kissel *et al.* [39] have produced perhaps the most detailed results for the shape function using relativistic partial-wave calculations. Although their results were limited to a few benchmark cases, the extension to other cases was suggested by an analytical parametrization in terms of Legendre polynomials. Acosta *et al.* [52] proposed a simpler parametrization based on a Lorentz-boosted dipole distribution,

$$
\begin{aligned}
S^{\mathrm{KQP}} = A\frac{3}{16\pi}&\left[1+\left(\frac{\cos\theta-\beta'}{1-\beta'\cos\theta}\right)^2\right]\frac{1-\beta'^2}{(1-\beta'\cos\theta)^2}\\
+ (1-A)\frac{3}{8\pi}&\left[1-\left(\frac{\cos\theta-\beta'}{1-\beta'\cos\theta}\right)^2\right]\frac{1-\beta'^2}{(1-\beta'\cos\theta)^2},
\end{aligned}\tag{3.7}
$$

with $\beta' = \beta_{\mathrm{i}}(1+B)$. The adjustable parameters A and B depend on (k, Z, E), and can be fitted to the benchmark results of Kissel *et al.* [39], or values calculated by the computer program BREMS [53], which implements the same theory. Note that this shape function (referred to as KQP in ref. [51]) is consistent with the calculations performed by Pratt *et al.* [45] for the electron-nucleus bremsstrahlung cross section differential in energy, which is included in the NIST cross-section database for energies below 2 MeV (see Section 3.2.1).

Besides the numerical results for the shape function obtained by calculations in partial-wave expansions, various analytical expressions derived in the Born approximation have been suggested. The review by Koch and Motz [13] included several analytical PWBA formulas for the electron-nucleus bremsstrahlung cross section double differential in photon energy and emission angle, developed in various approximations. These cross sections have been implemented in different Monte Carlo code systems for sampling of the bremsstrahlung angular distribution. It should be noted that the habitual practice has been to assume that the electron-electron bremsstrahlung angular distribution is the same as for electron-nucleus.

A commonly used double differential PWBA cross section formula is the 2BN (Born approximation, no screening) expression described by Koch and Motz,

$$
\begin{aligned}
\mathrm{d}^2\sigma_{\mathrm{br}}^{\mathrm{2BN}} =\ &\frac{\alpha Z^2 r_{\mathrm{e}}^2}{4\pi}\frac{\mathrm{d}k}{k}\frac{p'}{p}\frac{\mathrm{d}\hat{\boldsymbol{\Omega}}_\gamma}{\Delta_0^2}\left\{\frac{4(2E_{\mathrm{tot}}^2+1)\sin^2\theta}{p^2\Delta_0^2}\right.\\
&-\frac{5E_{\mathrm{tot}}^2+2E_{\mathrm{tot}}E_{\mathrm{tot}}'-2E_{\mathrm{tot}}'\Delta_0+3}{p^2}-\frac{p^2-k^2}{Q^2}\\
&+\frac{2L}{p^3p'}\left[\frac{E_{\mathrm{tot}}(3k-p^2E_{\mathrm{tot}}')\sin^2\theta}{\Delta_0^2}+E_{\mathrm{tot}}^2(E_{\mathrm{tot}}^2+E_{\mathrm{tot}}'^2-4)\right.\\
&\left.+E_{\mathrm{tot}}E_{\mathrm{tot}}'-\frac{E_{\mathrm{tot}}'^2}{2}+\frac{(k\Delta_0+1)}{2}(E_{\mathrm{tot}}^2+E_{\mathrm{tot}}E_{\mathrm{tot}}'-1)+1\right]\\
&\left.-\left(\frac{2\epsilon\Delta_0}{p'}\right)-\left(\frac{\epsilon^Q}{p'Q}\right)\left[\frac{k\Delta_0(p^2-k^2)}{Q^2}+3k\Delta_0-2\right]\right\},
\end{aligned}\tag{3.8}
$$

where α is the fine-structure constant, r_e is the classical electron radius, and

$$\Delta_0 = E_{\text{tot}}(1 - \beta_i \cos\theta), \qquad\qquad Q^2 = p^2 + k^2 - 2pk\cos\theta,$$

$$\epsilon = \ln\left(\frac{E'_{\text{tot}} + p'}{E'_{\text{tot}} - p'}\right), \qquad\qquad \epsilon^Q = \ln\left(\frac{Q + p'}{Q - p'}\right),$$

$$L = \ln\left(\frac{E_{\text{tot}} E'_{\text{tot}} - 1 + pp'}{E_{\text{tot}} E'_{\text{tot}} - 1 - pp'}\right),$$

with (E_{tot}, p) and (E'_{tot}, p') representing (total energy, momentum) of the electron prior to and after the bremsstrahlung emission, respectively. Note that Koch and Motz have in their formulations of the differential PWBA cross section expressed the electron and photon energies in units of the electron rest energy $(m_e c^2)$, and the momenta in units of $m_e c$.

The above expression for the double differential cross section was derived by Sauter [54] for bremsstrahlung in the electric field of a bare atomic nucleus, i.e., assuming no screening by the atomic electrons. Although it was derived without any restriction on the magnitude of the energy, scatter angle, and emission angle, it is inherently limited by the use of the PWBA theory. Recall that the first Born approximation makes the results less reliable for lower-energy electrons and higher-Z target materials. Nevertheless, for bremsstrahlung emission from a thick x-ray target (i.e., a typical x-ray tube anode), results obtained using 2BN have been shown to be in good agreement with more detailed partial-wave results [51].

The main practical drawback with 2BN is that it has a long functional form that is inefficient for some applications. A useful alternative, at high energies, is the 2BS (Born approximation, corrected for screening) double differential cross section described by Koch and Motz, which was derived by Schiff [55] for the bremsstrahlung emission in the electric field of a nucleus corrected (based on the Thomas-Fermi potential) for atomic electron screening effects,

$$d^2\sigma_{\text{br}}^{\text{2BS}} = 4\alpha Z^2 r_e^2 \frac{dk}{k} \frac{ydy}{(1 + y^2)^2} \left\{ \frac{16y^2 r}{(1 + y^2)^2} - (1 + r)^2 \right.$$
$$\left. - \left[\frac{4y^2 r}{(1 + y^2)^2} - (1 + r^2) \right] \ln M(y) \right\}, \qquad (3.9)$$

where

$$y = E_{\text{tot}}\theta, \quad r = \frac{E'_{\text{tot}}}{E_{\text{tot}}}, \quad \frac{1}{M(y)} = \left(\frac{k}{2E_{\text{tot}} E'_{\text{tot}}}\right)^2 + \left(\frac{Z^{1/3}}{111(1 + y^2)}\right)^2.$$

This expression was developed with extreme-relativistic and small-angle approximations, which limits its usefulness for lower energy applications.

Kawrakow *et al.* [34] have attempted to extend the applicability of 2BS, by noting that the angle-dependent leading term of 2BN $[(1 - \beta_i \cos\theta)^{-2}]$ and 2BS $[(1 + y^2)^{-2}]$ are, apart from a normalization factor, approximately equal for high energies and small angles. Hence, they implemented the intrinsic bremsstrahlung angular distribution by adapting the 2BS formula with the following modification to match the leading term of 2BN,

$$y^2 = \beta_{\mathrm{i}}(1 + \beta_{\mathrm{i}})E_{\mathrm{tot}}^2(1 - \cos\theta). \tag{3.10}$$

The resulting shape function (referred to as KM) allows for efficient sampling of θ using the method described by Bielajew *et al.* [56]. However, an even more efficient shape function was suggested, which consists of taking only the leading term of the 2BN formula,

$$S^{\mathrm{SIM}} = \Delta_0^{-2}\left(\int \frac{\mathrm{d}\hat{\Omega}_\gamma}{\Delta_0^2}\right)^{-1}, \tag{3.11}$$

where Δ_0 is defined on the previous page. Despite the relatively simple form, this shape function (referred to as SIM in ref. [51]) has been shown to perform well when calculating the bremsstrahlung emission from a thick x-ray target, especially for incident electron energies exceeding about 50 keV [51].

In addition to the above described detailed theories, a simplified approximation that has been assumed in analytical x-ray tube spectra models is that the bremsstrahlung shape function is uniform, $S^{\mathrm{UNI}} = 1/(4\pi)$ [28, 29, 57, 58]. This assumption stems from the rationale that the intrinsic bremsstrahlung angular distribution is masked by the diffuse directional distribution of multiple scattered electrons. However, a substantial amount of the bremsstrahlung that escapes the target is generated in the region before diffusion (i.e., the multiple-scattering region) [59]. Furthermore, even in the region of diffusion, the electrons retain a directional preference in that more electrons are forward scattered than backscattered. Therefore, adopting a uniform shape function can result in the emitted x-ray fluence being overestimated by up to 15% [51, 59].

3.3   CHARACTERISTIC X-RAY PRODUCTION

An x ray with characteristic energy is produced when an atom with a vacancy in one of its inner shells relaxes from its excited state through a radiative transition, that is, by *fluorescence*. In an x-ray tube anode, atomic shell vacancies are generated as a result of the following two types of particle-atom interactions (illustrated in fig. 3.1):

- Inner-shell impact ionization (si)—an electron penetrating the target knocks out an inner-shell electron in an inelastic hard collision

- Photon-atom interactions (ph)—a bound electron is ejected in a photoelectric absorption or Compton scattering of a bremsstrahlung photon generated by the deceleration of an electron penetrating the x-ray target

Since the two types of interaction processes producing fluorescence are fundamentally different in that they are initiated by charged (electrons) or uncharged (photons) particles, they produce distinctly different spatial distributions of x-ray fluorescence in the anode. This difference can be observed in figs. 3.7 and 3.8, which show the x-ray production as a function of the electron penetration depth in tungsten and molybdenum.

The depth distribution of x-ray fluorescence following ionization by electron impact resembles the depth distribution of the incident electrons penetrating into the target (see fig. 3.2). The production of fluorescence following impact ionization is limited to penetration depths where the electrons retain enough of the incident kinetic energy to overcome the inner-shell ionization threshold. In contrast, x-ray fluorescence following ionization initiated by photon interactions extends considerably deeper into the target due to the long mean free path length of bremsstrahlung photons. Notice that the K x-ray fluorescence following ionization by photon interactions is more prominent for tungsten than molybdenum, due to the greater photoelectric cross section and the reduced electron impact ionization cross section for higher-Z materials [61].

Although characteristic x rays may, under certain conditions, have an anisotropic intrinsic angular distribution (caused by the alignment of atomic hole states) [62], the emission of x rays within a typical target with randomly oriented atoms can be accurately described as isotropic. This means that the emission of characteristic radiation in an x-ray tube anode can be

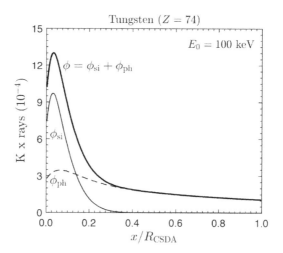

Figure 3.7: Depth distribution of x-ray fluorescence in tungsten per 100 keV incident electron. The figures show Monte Carlo-calculated number of K x rays produced following ionization by electron impact (ϕ_{si}) and photon interactions (ϕ_{ph}), differential in depth scaled by the electron CSDA range, $x/R_{\mathrm{CSDA}}(E_0)$; data extracted from ref. [60].

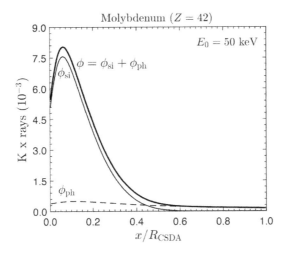

Figure 3.8: Depth distribution of x-ray fluorescence in molybdenum per 50 keV incident electron. The figures show Monte Carlo-calculated number of K x rays produced following ionization by electron impact (ϕ_{si}) and photon interactions (ϕ_{ph}), differential in depth scaled by the electron CSDA range, $x/R_{CSDA}(E_0)$; data extracted from ref. [60].

assumed to occur with no memory of the direction of motion of the particles that produced the atomic ionizations. The characteristic x-ray emission can therefore be fully described in terms of the spatial (depth) distribution of x-ray fluorescence in the target, combined with the specific transition probabilities and characteristic line energies of the target material.

Besides *radiative transitions* resulting in the emission of x rays, an excited ion can also relax through a *non-radiative transition*, that is, by the ejection of an atomic electron. The probability of a radiative transition (versus a competing non-radiative transition) is given by the *fluorescence yield*, which can be expressed as the sum of all radiative transition probabilities for a given shell S0,

$$\omega_{S0}(Z) = \sum_{S1} P_{S0-S1}(Z). \tag{3.12}$$

The summation extends over all subshells S1 from which electrons can transition to fill a vacancy in the inner-shell S0, for a target atom with atomic number Z. Hence, we may for a given radiative transition express the average number of x rays emitted per one fluorescence as,

$$v_{S0-S1}(Z) = P_{S0-S1}/\omega_{S0}(Z), \tag{3.13}$$

with characteristic energy that is the difference in binding energies between the final and initial shell,

$$k_{S0-S1} = U_{S0} - U_{S1}. \tag{3.14}$$

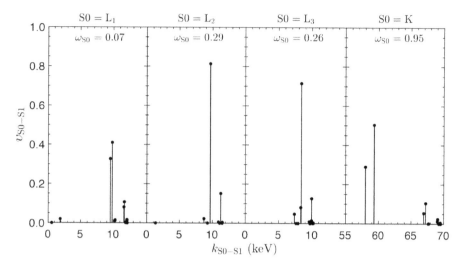

Figure 3.9: Radiative transition data (eqs. 3.12–3.14) for tungsten, extracted from the Livermore Evaluated Atomic Data Library (EPICS2017 version) [63].

The transition probabilities and emission energies for a given target material can, for instance, be found in the comprehensive and widely used Livermore EADL library. An example of such data for tungsten is presented in fig. 3.9, extracted from the most recent version of the Livermore EADL library (EPICS2017) [63].

A supplementary Python script to this chapter is available in the book's online software repository, at https://bitbucket.org/caxtus. The script is called *percent_char.py* and uses the SpekPy-v2 toolkit; it plots the percentage contribution of characteristic radiation to the total fluence as a function of tube potential. The tube filtration is set to 3 mm Be (inherent), 0.208 mm Al (added) and 500 mm of air (exit window to detector). Try increasing the filtration of aluminium to 1 mm. How do the results change and why?

CHAPTER 4

Basic dosimetry and beam-quality characterization

T HIS chapter provides the basic concepts and formulations entering into the determination of the absorbed dose to a patient or to any material exposed to a beam of x rays. Basic quantities of different types forming the basis of radiation dosimetry are defined. The various coefficients and factors necessary for the dosimetry of an x-ray spectrum are expressed in terms of parameters that represent the characteristics of the spectrum. These parameters provide the link between key data evaluated for mono-energetic photons and the necessary data for beam spectra generated by x-ray tubes.

4.1 FIELD AND DOSIMETRY QUANTITIES

Quantities that characterize a radiation field of charged or uncharged particles are presented first (Section 4.1.1). This is followed by a summary of the most important coefficients describing the transfer and deposition of energy to matter following the interactions of charged and uncharged particles (Section 4.1.2); it assumes the reader to be familiar with the most important interaction effects of radiation with matter. Finally, basic dosimetric quantities are defined and expressed in terms of the field quantities and interaction coefficients (Section 4.1.3).

4.1.1 Field quantities

A *radiation field* is a group of particles, that is, photons, electrons, positrons, protons, neutrons, etc., each having *radiant energy* and moving in a certain direction. Radiant energies exclude the particle rest energy. For particles with a mass, the radiant energy is the kinetic energy of the particle and the

DOI: 10.1201/9781003058168-4

symbol E is used throughout this book for electrons; the energy of photons is represented by the symbol k.

Given a radiation field consisting of N charged and/or uncharged particles, the field quantity *fluence* is defined by ICRU Report 85 [64] as the number of particles $\mathrm{d}N$ incident on a sphere of cross-sectional area $\mathrm{d}a$,

$$\Phi = \frac{\mathrm{d}N}{\mathrm{d}a}, \tag{4.1}$$

with unit cm^{-2}. The concept of a sphere conveys the idea of an area which is perpendicular to the direction of each particle, see fig. 4.1. In Monte Carlo calculations, the average fluence in a volume V is given by the sum of particle tracks within the volume, $\bar{\Phi} = \sum(\mathrm{d}\ell)/\mathrm{d}V$, occasionally referred to as *track-length fluence*.

Sometimes it is of interest to refer to the number of particles crossing a fixed plane in either direction, a quantity termed *planar fluence* which is defined as [65]

$$\Phi^{\mathrm{P}} = \frac{\mathrm{d}N}{\mathrm{d}a}\,\overline{\cos\theta_\Phi} = \Phi\,\overline{\cos\theta_\Phi}, \tag{4.2}$$

where θ is the angle between the direction of the exiting particles and their initial direction and $\overline{\cos\theta_\Phi}$ is the fluence-weighted mean value of the directional

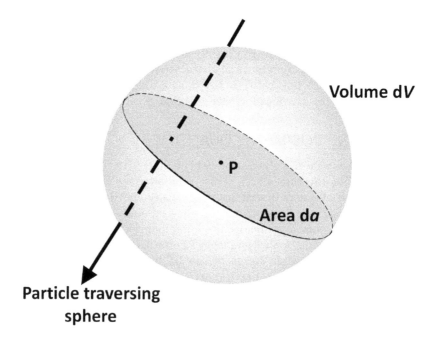

Figure 4.1: Characterizing the radiation field at a point P in terms of the particle trajectories traversing a sphere of cross section $\mathrm{d}a$ centred on P provides the definition of particle fluence.

cosine. Figure 4.2 illustrates the concept using a *thought experiment* in which all the particles in a plane-parallel beam scatter through the same angle.

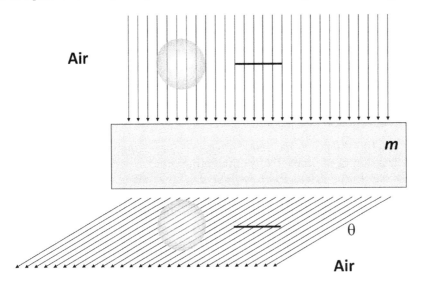

Figure 4.2: *Gedankenexperiment* illustrating a plane-parallel particle beam scattered in a slab of medium m through an angle θ. The number of particle tracks crossing a flat surface (planar fluence, Φ^{P}) is constant before and after scattering. However, for a spherical volume having the same cross-sectional area, the number of tracks (fluence, Φ) increases after scattering according to $\Phi = \Phi^{\mathrm{P}}/\cos\theta$.

A related field quantity is the *energy fluence*, defined as the radiant energy incident on a sphere of cross-sectional area $\mathrm{d}a$, which, for example for electrons, can be written as

$$\Psi = E\,\Phi, \tag{4.3}$$

with unit J cm^{-2}, where E is the electron radiant energy. The analogous expression for photons replaces E by k, that is, $\Psi = k\,\Phi$.

The field quantities fluence and energy fluence can be expressed as distributions with respect to energy, E or k, for electrons and photons, respectively, as

$$\Phi_E = \frac{\mathrm{d}\Phi}{\mathrm{d}E}\;; \qquad \Psi_E = \frac{\mathrm{d}\Psi}{\mathrm{d}E}\,, \tag{4.4}$$

where $\mathrm{d}\Phi$ is the fluence of electrons with energy between E and $E + \mathrm{d}E$ and $\mathrm{d}\Psi$ its energy fluence, and

$$\Phi_k = \frac{\mathrm{d}\Phi}{\mathrm{d}k}\;; \qquad \Psi_k = \frac{\mathrm{d}\Psi}{\mathrm{d}k}\,, \tag{4.5}$$

where $\mathrm{d}\Phi$ is the fluence of photons with energy between k and $k + \mathrm{d}k$ and $\mathrm{d}\Psi$ its energy fluence.

The two quantities differential in energy, Φ_E and Ψ_E, or Φ_k and Ψ_k, are commonly referred to as *fluence spectrum* and *energy-fluence spectrum*, respectively. Their respective integrals lead to the total quantities in terms of E or k, for electrons and photons, respectively. For the latter, they are

$$\Phi = \int_0^{k_{\max}} \Phi_k \, dk \; ; \qquad \Psi = \int_0^{k_{\max}} \Psi_k \, dk \; . \tag{4.6}$$

4.1.2 Interaction coefficients

For a photon fluence Φ incident on a given target material of density ρ, the mean fraction of photons dN/N interacting along a distance $d\ell$ in the target defines the *linear attenuation coefficient* μ. Its unit is cm^{-1}. The reciprocal of μ defines the *mean free path* or mean path length traversed by a photon between two consecutive interactions.[1] As inferred from its definition, the linear attenuation coefficient depends strongly on the mass density of the material, a constraint removed by the *mass attenuation coefficient*, μ/ρ, which is defined as

$$\frac{\mu}{\rho} = \frac{1}{\rho \, d\ell} \frac{dN}{N} \; , \tag{4.7}$$

with the unit of cm^2 g^{-1}. This is in fact the macroscopic equivalent of the total cross section for the different photon interaction modalities and can be written as

$$\frac{\mu}{\rho} = \frac{N_A}{M} \sum_j \sigma_j = \frac{n}{\rho} \sum_j \sigma_j \; , \tag{4.8}$$

where N_A is the Avogadro constant, M is the molar mass of the material, σ_j is the cross section for an interaction of the type j, and n is the number of target entities per volume.

An energy-related photon interaction coefficient is the *mass energy-transfer coefficient*, μ_{tr}/ρ, which accounts for the transfer of photon energy to the electrons produced in the different interactions. It is defined as

$$\frac{\mu_{tr}}{\rho} = \frac{N_A}{M} \sum_j f_j \sigma_j \; , \tag{4.9}$$

where, for each interaction type j, the coefficient f_j represents the mean fraction of the photon energy which is transferred to the kinetic energy of the electrons produced [65].

The amount of energy transferred which is deposited locally is given by the *mass energy-absorption coefficient*, μ_{en}/ρ. Depending on the photon energy,

---

[1] Note that the concepts of attenuation coefficient and mean free path can also be used for electrons, but the very large number of interactions occurring even in short distances makes their use impractical in most cases. One significant exception is in certain types of Monte Carlo procedures, see e.g. ref. [35].

a fraction of the energy transferred can escape the local volume; this is given by the *radiative fraction* g, defined as the fraction of the kinetic energy of the generated electrons which is lost in radiative processes such as bremsstrahlung, fluorescence, etc. The two-photon interaction coefficients are related by

$$\frac{\mu_{en}}{\rho} = \frac{\mu_{tr}}{\rho}(1-g), \tag{4.10}$$

and are typically given in cm^2 g^{-1}. They convey the concept of photons being particles whose energy deposition to matter is indirect[2], as secondary electrons are created first by photon interactions, they are given a certain amount of energy, and this energy is subsequently deposited in matter through successive electron interactions.

A comparison of the values of μ/ρ and μ_{en}/ρ (or μ_{tr}/ρ) for silicon is shown in fig. 4.3, along with the ratios of mass energy-absorption coefficients silicon-to-water between 1 and 300 keV. Note that the values of μ_{tr}/ρ are identical to those of μ_{en}/ρ in the energy interval of the figure.

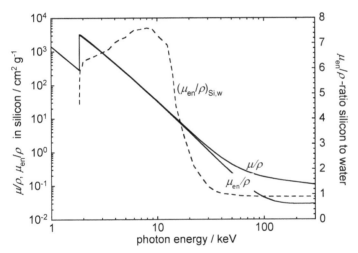

Figure 4.3: Values of μ/ρ and μ_{en}/ρ or μ_{tr}/ρ for silicon. Illustrated also are the ratios of mass energy-absorption coefficients silicon-to-water, $(\mu_{en}/\rho)_{Si,w}$.

For the electrons produced by photons, the extremely large number of interactions occurring in short distances lends itself to formulate interaction coefficients in terms of energy loss per unit path length. The *mass stopping power* S/ρ is defined by the mean energy lost by an electron while traversing a distance $d\ell$ in a material of density ρ; its unit is keV cm^2 g^{-1} when the energy loss is in keV. It consists of the *mass electronic stopping power* S_{el}/ρ,

---

[2]In some old publications it is stated that photons are "indirectly ionizing radiation", a misleading term because it is not the ionization what is indirect, but the energy transferred to matter.

accounting for the energy lost through interactions with atomic electrons which result in the ionization or excitation of the atom, and the *mass radiative stopping power* S_{rad}/ρ, describing the energy lost through the emission of electromagnetic radiation in the electric fields of atomic nuclei or electrons, that is, the interaction type known as *bremsstrahlung*,

$$\frac{S}{\rho} = \frac{S_{el}}{\rho} + \frac{S_{rad}}{\rho}. \tag{4.11}$$

A related coefficient is the *continuous-slowing-down range*, R_{CSDA}, which represents the average length travelled by an electron when it slows down from an initial energy E_0 to final energy close to zero. As energy loss is considered to be continuous, it can be written

$$R_{CSDA}(E_0) = \rho \int\limits_{0}^{E_0} \frac{dE}{S(E)}, \tag{4.12}$$

with the unit of g cm^{-2}. Due to multiple scattering effects, the path of an electron is always rather tortuous, particularly in heavy materials, yielding a depth of maximum penetration (often termed *mean forward range*) which is substantially smaller than the CSDA range [65].

4.1.3 Dosimetric quantities

The dosimetry of photons with energies up to about 300 keV is governed by the quantity *kerma*, which accounts for the transfer of the kinetic energy of photon-produced electrons to a volume of material. Kerma is the acronym for *kinetic energy released per unit mass* and has the unit of gray (Gy). It can be shown [65] that in a given medium, kerma is related to the field quantities fluence and energy fluence through

$$K = k\,\Phi_{med} \left[\frac{\mu_{tr}(k)}{\rho} \right]_{med} = \Psi_{med} \left[\frac{\mu_{tr}(k)}{\rho} \right]_{med}, \tag{4.13}$$

where k is the photon energy, Φ is the photon fluence in the medium, and μ_{tr}/ρ is the photon mass energy-transfer coefficient of the medium at the energy k. As stated in ICRU Report 85 [64], expressing kerma in terms of fluence or energy fluence illustrates that one can refer to the kerma for a specified material inside a different material. For example, *water kerma free-in-air* can be obtained using

$$K_w(air) = K_w^{air} = k\,\Phi_{air} \left[\frac{\mu_{tr}(k)}{\rho} \right]_w. \tag{4.14}$$

When only a fraction of the energy transferred to the volume under consideration is locally deposited, the *collision* (or *electronic*) *kerma* describes the component of the kerma resulting from such energy deposition

$$K_{col} = K\,(1 - g), \tag{4.15}$$

where g is the radiative fraction defined above. K_{col} can also be expressed in terms of fluence and energy fluence using eqs. (4.10) and (4.13):

$$K_{col} = k\,\Phi_{med}\left[\frac{\mu_{en}(k)}{\rho}\right]_{med} = \Psi_{med}\left[\frac{\mu_{en}(k)}{\rho}\right]_{med}. \qquad (4.16)$$

It should be emphasized that at the photon energies considered in this book, the radiative fraction is practically negligible for light materials and most human tissues. For example, for 300 keV the mean energy of Compton-produced electrons is about 80 keV, for which the radiation yields in water, air, muscle, and bone are within 0.05%–0.07%. Hence, it is reasonable to assume that $\mu_{en}/\rho = \mu_{tr}/\rho$ and $K = K_{col}$. Additionally, when *charge-particle equilibrium* exists, the absorbed dose in the medium, D, i.e., the sum of all the energy deposits (energy imparted) in a mass of matter dm divided by dm, is numerically equal to the kerma, see fig. 4.4. Hence,

$$D \overset{CPE}{=} K = k\,\Phi_{med}\left[\frac{\mu_{tr}(k)}{\rho}\right]_{med}$$
$$\overset{g\approx0}{=} k\,\Phi_{med}\left[\frac{\mu_{en}(k)}{\rho}\right]_{med}. \qquad (4.17)$$

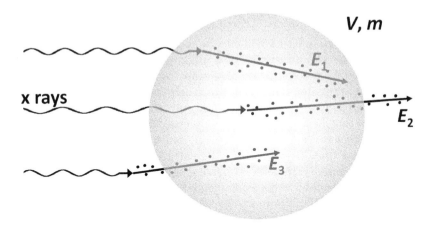

Figure 4.4: Distinction between absorbed dose D and kerma K with regard to a volume V of mass m. The kinetic energy of secondary electrons E_1 and E_2 contribute to K because both electrons are created inside V. The energy of electron E_3 does not contribute to K because is created outside V. Only the energy imparted (indicated by the dots) along the electron tracks inside V contribute to D. The absorbed dose will be equal to the kerma when the energy entering V is exactly equal to the energy leaving V, i.e., charged-particle equilibrium. Adapted from: Andreo *et al* 2017, figure 4.5, p. 233 [65]. Reproduced with permission of John Wiley & Sons.

The relationships above refer to mono-energetic photons. They can be generalized to a fluence spectrum or an energy-fluence spectrum of maximum photon energy k_{max} as

$$K = \int_0^{k_{max}} k\,[\Phi_k]_{med}\,[\mu_{en}(k)/\rho]_{med}\,dk$$

$$= \int_0^{k_{max}} [\Psi_k]_{med}\,[\mu_{en}(k)/\rho]_{med}\,dk. \tag{4.18}$$

A number of specific dosimetric quantities mostly intended for use with clinical equipment have been given by ICRU Report 74 [66] and IAEA TRS-457 [67] for diagnostic and interventional radiology, all based on an initial air kerma determination. A reference air kerma free-in-air is measured using a detector calibration coefficient $N_{K,air}$, which enters into subsequent definitions of the quantities. Examples include the incident air kerma, the entrance-surface air kerma, the air kerma-area product, air kerma-length product, the CT air kerma index, etc. Details can be found in the ICRU and IAEA references cited.

4.2   BEAM-QUALITY CHARACTERIZATION

Photon spectra given in terms of fluence or energy fluence are the most suitable descriptors of the characteristics of a photon beam, and expressions like eq. (4.18) enable the determination of relevant dosimetric quantities. However, detailed spectra are often not available or their use is not practical in routine work. Simpler calculated or experimental parameters have been developed over the years that have become widely accepted by the x-ray community to characterize the so-called *beam quality* and will be described in this section. It is emphasized that, as stressed in the early ICRU Report 10b [68] from the 1960s, one single parameter is not enough to characterize properly an x-ray beam. Unfortunately, this recommendation has not been followed widely. The more recent ICRU Report 74 [66] emphasized this constraint providing examples and suggestions that involved the use of two or three parameters.

4.2.1   Mean energy and coefficients

When the photon spectral distribution is available, either by measurement or by calculation, a commonly used parameter to characterize the quality of an x-ray beam is the *mean energy* of the spectrum. This is, however, not a unique specifier and has certain weaknesses. Firstly, it is possible for two different spectra to have identical or very similar mean energy. Secondly, and more important, depending on the type of spectrum available, given in terms of fluence or of energy fluence, the mean energy is defined differently.

The field quantity in which a spectrum is given should always be stated. Hence, for a fluence spectrum, the *fluence-weighted mean energy* is defined as

$$
\bar{k}_\Phi = \frac{\int\limits_0^{k_{\max}} k\Phi_k \, dk}{\int\limits_0^{k_{\max}} \Phi_k \, dk} \, , \tag{4.19}
$$

which is the ratio of total energy-fluence to total fluence, Ψ/Φ. For an energy-fluence spectrum, the *energy-fluence-weighted mean energy* is

$$
\bar{k}_\Psi = \frac{\int\limits_0^{k_{\max}} k\Psi_k \, dk}{\int\limits_0^{k_{\max}} \Psi_k \, dk} = \frac{\int\limits_0^{k_{\max}} k^2 \Phi_k \, dk}{\int\limits_0^{k_{\max}} k\Phi_k \, dk} \, . \tag{4.20}
$$

Note that the international standard ISO 437-1 [69] defines the *mean photon energy* according to eq. (4.19).

In radiation protection and diagnostic and interventional radiology applications, a third option has become frequently used, particularly at standards dosimetry laboratories [70]. The mean energy is stated in terms of air kerma, so that in analogy with $\bar{k}_\Phi$ and $\bar{k}_\Psi$ above, the *air-kerma-weighted mean energy* is defined as

$$
\bar{k}_{K_{\text{air}}} = \frac{\int\limits_0^{k_{\max}} k\, K_{\text{air},k} \, dk}{\int\limits_0^{k_{\max}} K_{\text{air},k} \, dk}
$$

$$
= \frac{\int\limits_0^{k_{\max}} k^2 \Phi_{k,\text{air}} \, [\mu_{\text{en}}(k)/\rho]_{\text{air}} \, dk}{\int\limits_0^{k_{\max}} k\, \Phi_{k,\text{air}} \, [\mu_{\text{en}}(k)/\rho]_{\text{air}} \, dk} \, , \tag{4.21}
$$

where $K_{\text{air},k}$ is referred to as the *air kerma spectrum*, obtained at each energy k by calculation from Φ_k or Ψ_k distributions. The air-kerma-weighted mean energy $\bar{k}_{K_{\text{air}}}$ is often referred to as the *dose-weighted mean energy*, simply denoted by $\bar{k}_D$ or $\bar{k}_{D_{\text{air}}}$. It should be emphasized however that, as can be seen in eq. (4.21), this modality of mean energy depends on the data set selected for the mass energy-absorption coefficients of air, for which no international recommendations have been made so far, see ICRU Report 90 [44]. The $\bar{k}_{K_{\text{air}}}$ modality can then be said to be less robust than $\bar{k}_\Phi$ and $\bar{k}_\Psi$.

To illustrate the difference between the various options used for representing x-ray spectra and their influence on the respective mean energy, fig. 4.5 shows distributions differential in energy for a 135 kV x-ray spectrum in terms

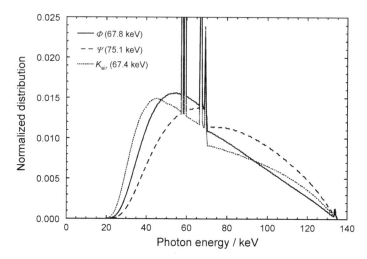

Figure 4.5: Fluence Φ (solid line), energy fluence Ψ (dashed line), and air kerma K_{air} (dotted line) spectra for the same 135 kV x-ray beam; the corresponding mean energies are given in the data symbols within parentheses. The three distributions are normalized to their respective integral and the heights of the fluorescent lines in the figure have been limited for clarity.

of fluence, energy fluence, and air kerma, where the three spectra correspond to the same x-ray beam.

Mean energy is often used to obtain from a lookup table a mean interaction coefficient which is assumed to correspond to the spectrum at hand, e.g., $\mu(\bar{k}_\Psi)$ for the lineal attenuation coefficient of the energy-fluence-weighted mean energy. An accurate mean coefficient value should, however, be obtained by weighting $\mu(k)$ values with the detailed spectrum, which results in the *energy-fluence-weighted average coefficient*

$$
\bar{\mu}_\Psi = \frac{\int\limits_0^{k_{max}} \mu(k)\,\Psi_k\,\mathrm{d}k}{\int\limits_0^{k_{max}} \Psi_k\,\mathrm{d}k} \ , \tag{4.22}
$$

usually different from $\mu(\bar{k}_\Psi)$. Similar mean coefficient values can be formulated and conclusions drawn for $\mu_{en}(\bar{k}_\Psi)/\rho$ and $\overline{(\mu_{en}/\rho)}_\Psi$, or for $\mu_{en}(\bar{k}_\Phi)/\rho$ and the *fluence-weighted average coefficient* $\overline{(\mu_{en}/\rho)}_\Phi$, etc.

To illustrate the differences between parameter values obtained from different types of spectra and between the methods to evaluate mean values of coefficients, an example case has been developed whose results are given in table 4.1. The fluence spectrum corresponds to a 30 kV x-ray beam, filtered by 3 mm of beryllium, 0.208 mm of aluminium, and 500 mm of air, and has been calculated with SpekPy-v2 [71]. The energy-fluence and the air kerma spectra are calculated using eqs. (4.3) and (4.18), respectively. Starting with mean energies ranging from 13 keV to 18 keV approximately, substantial differences can be seen between the different columns and row pairs that will affect the output of most calculations based on these parameters, such as kerma or beam attenuation in any medium. To avoid ambiguities, the type of spectral distribution used in any calculation should always be stated.

4.2.2 Half-value layer

The quality of an x-ray beam is most often characterized through suitable attenuation measurements in a given material, usually aluminium and copper. For this purpose, the air kerma of x rays transmitted by different thicknesses of the selected material is measured under narrow-beam geometry conditions, normalizing the results to the air kerma measured without attenuation material. The "HVL" can also be determined by calculation when the incident spectrum is known, e.g. using an iterative procedure. Material thicknesses corresponding to different attenuation fractions define n-value layers.

The *first half-value layer*, HVL_1, is defined as the thickness of material required to reduce the air kerma to 50% of its initial value without attenuation material. The *second half-value layer*, HVL_2, is the additional material thickness necessary to reduce the initial air kerma to 25% of the initial value. For x-ray beams below about 100 kV, HVLs are typically expressed in millimetres of high-purity aluminium; above 100 kV, HVLs are usually given in millimetres of high-purity copper. There is a region of overlap around 100 kV where HVLs can be given in thickness of any of the two materials. The ratio HVL_1/HVL_2 defines the *homogeneity index* h_i, which provides a sense of the spectral width and is unity for mono-energetic photons.

The first half-value layer in aluminium or copper is probably the most widely used single x-ray beam quality specifier, frequently shortened to half-value layer. It has been shown, however, that x-ray beams generated with different tube potential and/or filtration may have the same HVL, rendering the use of this single parameter non-rigorous. Illustrative examples are shown in ref. [65] and in ICRU Report 74 [66]. The latter suggests using the combination of tube potential, HVL_1 and HVL_2, which is equivalent to including the homogeneity index in the beam quality specification given as the triplet (kV, HVL_1, h_i), although for most practical dosimetry purposes the pair (kV, HVL_1) is suitable for the beam quality specification of x-ray beams.

In radiation shielding applications, the use of the *tenth-value layer*, TVL, is rather common. Its definition follows that of the HVL but in this case, the air kerma is reduced to one-tenth of its initial value without attenuation material.

A related quantity used in x-ray beam quality specification is the *effective energy*, defined as the energy of a mono-energetic photon having the same

Table 4.1: Parameters obtained from different types of spectral distributions and mean coefficient values from different evaluation methods for a 30 kV x-ray spectrum.

Spectral distribution:	fluence (Φ_k)	energy-fluence (Ψ_k)	air kerma ($K_{air,k}$)
Mean energy, k_{mean} (keV)	$\bar{k}_\Phi = 16.65$	$\bar{k}_\Psi = 18.38$	$\bar{k}_{K_{air}} = 13.11$
$(\mu_{en}/\rho)_{air}$ from k_{mean} (cm^2 g^{-1})	$\mu_{en}[\bar{k}_\Phi]/\rho = 0.937$	$\mu_{en}[\bar{k}_\Psi]/\rho = 0.687$	$\mu_{en}[\bar{k}_{K_{air}}]/\rho = 1.985$
$(\mu_{en}/\rho)_{air}$ from spectrum (cm^2 g^{-1})	$\overline{(\mu_{en}/\rho)}_\Phi = 1.910$	$\overline{(\mu_{en}/\rho)}_\Psi = 1.361$	$\overline{(\mu_{en}/\rho)}_{K_{air}} = 3.456$
$(\mu/\rho)_{air}$ from k_{mean} (cm^2 g^{-1})	$\mu[\bar{k}_\Phi]/\rho = 1.203$	$\mu[\bar{k}_\Psi]/\rho = 0.941$	$\mu[\bar{k}_{K_{air}}]/\rho = 2.296$
$(\mu/\rho)_{air}$ from spectrum (cm^2 g^{-1})	$\overline{(\mu/\rho)}_\Phi = 2.200$	$\overline{(\mu/\rho)}_\Psi = 1.632$	$\overline{(\mu/\rho)}_{K_{air}} = 3.796$

HVL_1 as the beam whose quality is to be specified [69]. The effective energy does not provide more information than HVL_1, but can be useful to describe a heavily filtered beam with a spectrum approaching the shape of a mono-energetic beam [65]. Note that its precise value does depend on whether the HVL_1 value is specified in aluminium or copper.

A supplementary Python script to this chapter is available in the book's online software repository, at https://bitbucket.org/caxtus. The script is called *mean_coeff.py* and uses the SpekPy-v2 toolkit; it reproduces the data of table 4.1. Try increasing the aluminium filtration to 1 mm and running the script. Do the coefficients calculated via the fluence, energy-fluence and kerma spectra agree more or less closely after the increase in filtration? Can you explain this? Note that the script also prints out the homogeneity index, h_i.

II

Modelling

CHAPTER 5

A review of analytical models for the x-ray spectrum

NALYTICAL models are empirical, semi-empirical, or entirely theoretical models for predicting x-ray spectra, that, unlike the Monte Carlo method, do not use random sampling. This chapter summarizes some landmarks from a century of developments and takes a closer look at some of the models.

5.1 KRAMERS AND THE EARLY 1920S

By the early 1920s, 25 years after their discovery, x rays were being used worldwide in a range of applications. X-ray tube technology had also advanced and was continuing apace. Theoretical models for predicting spectra lagged behind. To understand the challenges, it is important to understand some context.

That the *cathode rays* used to produce x rays were particles, was only demonstrated in 1897, the discovery of these *electrons* credited to Thomson [72]. Yet little was known about the interactions of electrons with matter. In 1912, Whiddington published measurements of the speed of electrons transmitted through films. He determined the empirical relationship [73],

$$\beta^4 = \beta_0^4 - ax. \tag{5.1}$$

where β_0 is the incident speed of the electron (in units of c, the speed of light), x is the thickness of the film, β is the mean speed of the electrons on their exit and a is a constant. This result agreed with theoretical predictions made by Thomson based on some simple assumptions [74]. At the weakly relativistic speeds investigated by Whiddington ($\beta_0 < 0.3$), the empirical result can also

DOI: 10.1201/9781003058168-5

be reformulated as,

$$E^2 = E_0^2 - bx \tag{5.2}$$

where $E_0 \ (= mc^2\beta_0^2/2$ with m the electron mass) is the incident kinetic energy of the electrons, E is the mean energy of the electrons on exit and b is a constant. The result, in either form, has become known as the Whiddington or Thomson-Whiddington relation. Note that according to the relation, the mean energy loss per thickness penetrated is,

$$-\frac{\mathrm{d}E}{\mathrm{d}x} = \frac{b}{2E} \text{ or } \frac{b}{mc^2\beta^2}, \tag{5.3}$$

In 1913, Bohr presented a landmark classical and non-relativistic result for the energy-loss of charged particles in matter, informed by the emerging field of quantum physics [75]. Applying it to electrons, the classical result for collision (electronic) stopping power can be expressed as,

$$-\frac{\mathrm{d}E}{\mathrm{d}x} = 4\pi mc^2 r_e^2 \frac{nZ}{\beta^2} \ln\left(\frac{K\hbar c\beta^3}{r_e I}\right) \tag{5.4}$$

where n is atomic density, Z is the material atomic number, I is the mean excitation energy of the target atoms, $\hbar$ is the reduced Planck constant, r_e is the classical electron radius and K is a constant taking a value of approximately 1.1. Over a limited energy range, the logarithmic term can be considered a constant. The Bohr formula therefore approximately reproduces the Whiddington relation, with,

$$b = 4\pi m^2 c^4 r_e^2 nZ \ln\left(\frac{K\hbar c\beta^3}{r_e I}\right) \equiv nZfL. \tag{5.5}$$

where L is the logarithmic term and $f = 4\pi m^2 c^4 r_e^2$ is independent of incident electron energy and the material.

This argument glosses over some important details, such as the assumption that the electrons penetrate into a material without deflection. In addition, even for non-relativistic energies, Bohr's classical result is never accurate for lighter charged particles such as electrons. Although Bohr had recently proposed the quantization of atomic energy levels [76] and Einstein had proposed the quantum nature of radiation a decade before [77], the insights of Heisenberg and others were still a few years away. In 1913, no consistent frameworks for quantum mechanical calculations had yet been elaborated and a rigorous quantum mechanical calculation had to wait.

Some remarkable discoveries regarding x-ray emissions had been made in the early twentieth century, despite a lack of a suitable theoretical framework and primitive equipment. Barkla had inferred the partial polarization of x-ray beams as early as 1905 [78, 79]. In the same work, he demonstrated the existence of characteristic radiation, even without a means of determining their energy. He later distinguished and named the K-series and L-series. As stated in his Nobel Prize lecture (3 June 1920) [80]: *"Each element when traversed by X-rays emits X-radiations characteristic of the element ... its quality is independent of that of the exciting primary radiation."*

The nature of bremsstrahlung in an x-ray tube was still mysterious. Although the radiative emissions of accelerating charges were well-understood within the context of classical electrodynamics, the importance of quantum physics was unclear. An initial (incorrect) suggestion, applying quantum concepts to bremsstrahlung, was that an electron of specific energy interacting in matter should also produce an x ray of specific energy, similar to Barkla's characteristic radiation [81].

Understanding the emissions from x-ray tubes were, in the early days, hampered by the limitations of the primitive Crookes tube and the lack of a method to investigate the energy of the emissions. In the decade preceding the 1920s, these issues were solved with the improvement of techniques for producing high vacuum, the introduction of the Coolidge hot-cathode tubes, and the invention of the ionization spectrometer by Bragg [81].

From 1915, more extensive and accurate measurements were being made. The interpretations of observations were still debated in 1920. While the quantization of atomic energy levels was well-appreciated, Barkla could still claim in his Nobel speech that: *"All this evidence seems to indicate that a quantum of radiation in the sense in which it has frequently been used, i.e. as an indivisible bundle of radiation energy, does not exist."*

Others appreciated that the presence of a maximum energy of x-ray emission proportional to voltage, as recognized by Duane and Hunt [82], suggested the quantum nature of the radiation and that the continuous x-ray spectra suggested that an electron could give up a varying fraction of its energy in x-ray emission. A good summary of the state of the field is presented in *The Bulletin of the National Research Council* from the period (Vol 1, Parts 6 and 7, 1920) [83].

By the early 1920s, it had been established empirically that the x-ray intensity spectrum from a thick target (after correction for absorption within the target) approximately follows the relation,

$$
\begin{aligned}
I_k^{\mathrm{emp}} &= \mathcal{A} \, Z \, (Ve - k) \text{ when k} < \text{Ve} \\
&= 0 \qquad\qquad\quad \text{otherwise}
\end{aligned}
\tag{5.6}
$$

where Z is the atomic number, V is the tube potential, e is the charge of an electron, k is the energy of x-ray emission and $\mathcal{A}$ is an experimentally-derived constant. At the time, small corrections were suggested to better fit experiments in the high-energy tip [84, 85], although later measurements questioned their necessity [86]. Despite the challenges of the emerging quantum theory of radiation, shouldn't an empirical result as simple as eq. (5.6) be deducible from a simple theory?

Developments were given impetus in 1923. That year, Kramers published an article, communicated to the journal *Philosophical Magazine* by no less than Bohr, entitled, *On the theory of X-ray absorption and of the continuous X-ray spectrum* [87]. He adopted a classical approach to the derivation of the frequency distribution of x-ray emissions and then interpreted the result from the perspective of quantum theory using the *correspondence principle*, i.e. the principle that in an appropriate limit the quantum prediction should reduce to the classical result. In particular, Kramers assumed:

- The electrons move non-relativistically

- On average, they radiate only a small portion of their energy

- Classically, the trajectory of an electron encountering a target nuclei follows a classical Kepler orbit

- The orbit for a substantial deflection can be approximated by a parabolic orbit i.e. the unbound orbit of maximum deflection

- The radiative emissions of a given frequency, ν, follow the prediction of classical electromagnetism for an electron following the trajectory

Kramers then applied the quantum mechanical interpretation that each frequency corresponds to the emission of x-ray quanta of corresponding energy, $k = h\nu$, and that the maximum emission energy was determined by Ve. Kramers' final thin-target cross section is,

$$\left(\frac{\mathrm{d}\sigma_{\mathrm{br}}}{\mathrm{d}k}\right)^{\mathrm{Kr}} = \frac{16\pi mc}{3\sqrt{3}\hbar}r_{\mathrm{e}}^3\frac{Z^2}{k\beta_{\mathrm{i}}^2}, \tag{5.7}$$

where β_i is the speed of the electron prior to bremsstrahlung emission. Note that the equation contains the same factor $(Z^2/k\beta_{\mathrm{i}}^2)$ present in eqs. 3.1 and 3.2, with the associated scaled cross section (χ) taking a constant value in Kramers' approximation.

The radiated energy per incident electron in a thin foil or thickness Δx is $k(\mathrm{d}\sigma/\mathrm{d}k)n\Delta x$. Inputting Kramers' cross section, we find that this energy is independent of the x-ray energy, k. The flatness of the thin-target intensity spectrum predicted by Kramers has been subsequently verified as approximately correct [88].

To obtain a thick target result, Kramers made use of the Whiddington relation, assuming that

$$E^2(x) = E_0^2 - nZfLx, \tag{5.8}$$

with L estimated by Kramers to take a value around 6. Kramers made the ansatz that the Whiddington relation represents the energy of an electron at depth x in a thick target. The maximum depth at which an x-ray of energy k can be emitted is then, $x_{\max} = (E_0^2 - k^2)/nZfL$. Assuming that emission is isotropic and measured at a distance r, using eq. (5.8) and integrating over eq. (5.7),

$$
\begin{aligned}
I_k^{\mathrm{Kr}} &= \frac{1}{4\pi r^2} \int_0^\infty k \left(\frac{\mathrm{d}\sigma_{br}}{\mathrm{d}k}\right)^{\mathrm{Kr}} n \,\mathrm{d}x \\
&= \frac{1}{4\pi r^2} \int_0^{x_{\max}} \left(\frac{16\pi mc}{3\sqrt{3}\hbar} r_e^3 \frac{Z^2}{\beta^2}\right) n \,\mathrm{d}x \\
&= \frac{1}{4\pi r^2} \int_k^{Ve} \left(\frac{8\pi m^2 c^3}{3\sqrt{3}\hbar} r_e^3 \frac{Z^2}{E}\right) n \left(\frac{\mathrm{d}E}{\mathrm{d}x}\right)^{-1} \mathrm{d}E \\
&= \frac{1}{4\pi r^2} \frac{8\pi m^2 c^3}{3\sqrt{3}\hbar} r_e^3 Z^2 n \int_k^{Ve} \frac{1}{E} \left(\frac{nZfL}{2E}\right)^{-1} \mathrm{d}E \\
&= \frac{1}{4\pi r^2} \frac{8\pi m^2 c^3}{3\sqrt{3}\hbar} r_e^3 \frac{2Z}{fL} \int_k^{Ve} \mathrm{d}E \\
&\equiv \frac{1}{4\pi r^2} \mathcal{B} Z \left(Ve - k\right),
\end{aligned}
\tag{5.9}
$$

where

$$
\mathcal{B} \equiv \frac{8\pi m^2 c^3}{3\sqrt{3}\hbar} r_e^3 \frac{2}{fL} = \frac{4}{3\sqrt{3}c\hbar} r_e \frac{1}{L}
\tag{5.10}
$$

and according to Kramers' work, is approximately 1.8×10^{-6} keV^{-1}. This Kramers-Whiddington formula is identical to the empirical result quoted in eq. (5.6), if the empirical constant $\mathcal{A}$ is equated with $\mathcal{B}/4\pi r^2$. Both the dependence on x-ray emission energy and on atomic number, as well as the absence of a dependence on atomic density, is reproduced.

To use Kramers' thick-target result in practice, we must account for the filtration of an x-ray tube. Following the Beer-Lambert law, this can be achieved by adding a suitable exponential term, $H(k)$. In addition, throughout this book, we typically express the x-ray spectrum in terms of the fluence spectrum, Φ_k. The intensity spectrum, I_k, is related to the energy-fluence rate. Converting from an intensity (expressed per incident electron) to fluence (per incident electron) and adding an exponential term, we find that Kramers-Whiddington thick target spectrum result becomes,

$$
\Phi_k^{\mathrm{Kr}} = \frac{1}{4\pi r^2} H(k) \mathcal{B} Z \frac{(Ve - k)}{k}.
\tag{5.11}
$$

For a single filter material, $H(k) = \exp\left[-\mu(k)t\right]$, with $\mu(k)$ the energy-dependent linear attenuation coefficient for the filtration material of thickness t.

The Kramers-Whiddington model has been widely used and referenced in the century following its publication. Its use has always had to contend with two fundamental deficiencies. Firstly, it is non-relativistic: the thin-target result on which it is based loses validity at higher tube potentials of around 50 kV. Secondly, it does not account for self-filtration of the emitted x rays by the target material itself.

5.2 THE NEXT 50 YEARS

From 1925, calculation frameworks emerged initially for non-relativistic and then relativistic quantum mechanics, through the work of a host of celebrated names too numerous to discuss here. In the ensuing decades, various calculations of the electron stopping power and bremsstrahlung cross section were made, valid in varying limits and approximations.

5.2.1 Collision stopping power

Quantum mechanical calculations for collision (electronic) stopping power began to emerge from the 1930s, beginning with Bethe [89,90] and Bloch [91, 92]. In the non-relativistic region, applying Bethe's formula to electrons, we find,

$$S_{el} = -\frac{dE}{dx} = 4\pi mc^2 r_e^2 \frac{nZ}{\beta^2} \ln\left(\frac{2mc^2\beta^2}{I}\right), \tag{5.12}$$

where x should properly be interpreted as the path length of the electron.

This formula has been used in many simple models for electron penetration into x-ray targets, often with the non-relativistic substitution of E for $\frac{1}{2}m\beta^2c^2$ [93]. While such results might be sufficient for heuristic purposes, for developing semi-empirical models, we emphasize that, the Bethe formula is not accurate for light particles like electrons, even for non-relativistic energies. Various corrections must be considered and the precise form of the collision stopping-power formula for electrons is rather complicated. We will not attempt a summary of the developments building on Bethe's result and refer the reader to comprehensive sources, such as Bohr's classic review [94], ICRU Report 37 [95], or textbooks [65,96]. However, the full relativistic result can be expressed as:

$$S_{el} = 2\pi mc^2 r_e^2 \frac{nZ}{\beta^2} \left[\ln\left(\frac{E^2}{I^2}\right) + \ln\left(1 + \frac{\tau}{2}\right) + F^-(\tau) - \delta\right], \tag{5.13}$$

where $\tau = E/mc^2$, δ is the density-effect correction and

$$F^-(\tau) = (1 - \beta^2)\left[1 + \tau^2/8 - (2\tau + 1)\ln 2\right] \tag{5.14}$$

The full formula does not lend itself to incorporation in simple models in the manner of the Whiddington relation, or even the non-relativistic Bethe formula. Tabulations, however, are straightforward to apply in computer programs implementing analytical models.

5.2.2 Bremsstrahlung cross sections

A summary of the various bremsstrahlung cross section formulas and their regions of applicability can be found in the celebrated review by Koch and

Motz [13] and the work of Seltzer and Berger [40, 43]. A few of the most important results are summarized in table 5.1.

The work of Sommerfeld [97] was a landmark and highly accurate within its limits. However, due to the complicated form of the results (in terms of hypergeometric functions) and its strictly non-relativistic validity, it has not been widely used in modelling x-ray tubes in the kilovoltage range.

The so-called Davies-Bethe-Maximon-Olsen (DBMO) result [40] forms the basis of cross sections widely used in the high megavoltage range, but again it is not applicable to the moderately relativistic energies corresponding to kilovoltage x-ray tubes.

A relativistic quantum mechanical calculation of bremsstrahlung was performed by Bethe and Heitler [46] and their result forms the backbone of most theoretical treatments using analytical formulae, outside of the extreme relativistic limit. The calculation was made in the plane-wave Born approximation, for electrons scattering from a bare nucleus. This is referred to as "BN" in Koch and Motz's nomenclature (Born and non-screened).

However, the plane-wave Born approximation used by Bethe and Heitler is only valid when [13]:

$$\frac{2\pi Z}{137\beta_i} << 1 \quad \text{and} \quad \frac{2\pi Z}{137\beta_f} << 1, \tag{5.15}$$

where β_i and β_f are the speed of the electron before and after bremsstrahlung emission, respectively, as a fraction of the speed of light. As can be seen, the Born approximation can be expected to break down for high-Z elements and low electron energies, which is precisely the conditions that are typically of interest for modelling x-ray tubes. Fortunately, an approximate correction due to Elwert [98] for the distortion of the plane wave by the Coulomb field of the nucleus (i.e. Coulomb correction), is available in the kilovoltage energy range.

The Bethe and Heitler result is also non-screened, that is, the nucleus is treated as bare, not clothed in electrons. The region of applicability for this approximation in the keV energy range is roughly [13]:

$$\frac{mc^2}{k} << \frac{137}{Z^{1/3}}. \tag{5.16}$$

This condition is fulfilled in many circumstances of interest to modelling x-ray tubes, but its applicability increasingly limited for higher Z materials and it always breaks down for sufficiently soft emissions. Screening corrections applicable to Bethe and Heitler have been estimated and are discussed in Koch and Motz review and Seltzer and Berger's work.

At the end of the period under discussion, in the early 1970s, more accurate partial-wave calculations were starting to become available, primarily through the work of Pratt and coworkers [99]. Such calculations become increasingly impractical for electron energies above 2 MeV, but that limit is perfectly sufficient for the energy range of x-ray tubes. Unfortunately, extensive tabulations did not become available until around 1980 [45, 100], when corresponding bremsstrahlung shape functions (angular distributions) were also published [39].

Table 5.1: A summary of key quantum mechanical calculations for bremsstrahlung emission. E is the kinetic energy of the electron prior to the bremsstrahlung emission. Note that Elwert's coulomb correction [98] may be applied to Bethe-Heitler's result.

Theory	Energy range	Screening correction	Coulomb correction
Sommerfeld (1931) (Dipole approx.) [97]	Non relativistic ($E < 50$ keV)	No	Yes
Bethe-Heitler (1934) (Born approx.) [46]	Relativistic (all E)	No	No
DBMO (1950s) (Born+corrections) [40]	Extreme relativistic ($E > 50$ MeV)	Yes	Yes
Pratt *et al* (1970s) (Partial wave) [100]	Relativistic ($E < 2$ MeV)	Yes	Yes

5.2.3 State-of-the-art in 1970

Dyson gives an excellent summary of the attempts to build semi-empirical models of bremsstrahlung and characteristic x-ray emissions up until 1970 [93]. The approaches often made use of simple results such as those presented in Section 5.1, as well as Bethe's formula. Yet, as previously observed, the use of the Whiddington relation—eq. (5.8)—is questionable and even Bethe's result—eq. (5.12)—is inaccurate for electrons. Kramers' thin-target bremsstrahlung cross section—eq. (5.7)—is also of limited validity. As we have seen, more accurate results for both electron collision stopping power and the bremsstrahlung cross section were available by 1970, albeit at the cost of adding complexity. Even so, a further difficulty had to be faced. Nothing described so far accounts for the random deflections of the electrons due to multiple-elastic scattering, the statistical nature of energy-loss, or the substantial fraction of electrons backscattered out of the target. In 1970 then, how would a scientist have best gone about estimating thick target bremsstrahlung?

Berger and Seltzer's [101] answer was to use a technique for radiation transport calculations developed at Los Alamos in the 1940s: the Monte Carlo method. Their computer code for thick target bremsstrahlung simulated electron and photon interactions, sampling from the relevant probability distributions. For high statistical certainty, the histories of a large number of incident electrons need to be simulated. As the code was developed for the specific task, Berger and Seltzer could include a number of optimizations to speed up calculations. Berger and Seltzer state that a computation took around 30 min on an IBM 360/91 computer for each incident electron energy. This is impressive, given the computational power of the day, but still rather slow.

The bremsstrahlung cross sections used in the Monte Carlo program were based on the Bethe-Heitler formula with screening and Coulomb corrections. The emphasis was on calculations for MeV electrons, but some results were presented for sub-MeV energies relevant to x-ray tubes also. Berger and Seltzer state [101]: *"The principal uncertainty in such calculations comes from a lack of sufficiently accurate bremsstrahlung cross sections, particularly for media of high atomic number and electron energies between 0.1 and 2 MeV, for which the cross section uncertainties may be as high as 20-30%."*

Applied scientists typically want simple and quick predictions of x-ray tube spectra, with a minimum of parameters to select. Highly accurate predictions may be worth waiting for, but predictions with high uncertainties are not. In 1970, Berger and Seltzer's code was state-of-the-art. But many scientists using tungsten target x-ray tubes needed something different. Considerable effort was put in to develop analytical models that overcame the limitations of the Kramers-Whiddington model and the impracticality of a full Monte Carlo treatment.

5.3   ANALYTICAL MODELS: 1970 UNTIL NOW

Analytical models can be empirical, semi-empirical, or entirely theoretical. It is not always unambiguous which of the three categories a model should be assigned to. The semi-empirical model, however, encapsulates the idea of splitting the calculation of x-ray emission into electron transport and emission parts, with an emphasis in obtaining results that fit measurements rather than theoretical rigour. Typically, the x-ray emission cross sections or the electron transport, or both, have empirically derived coefficients or values.

For the purpose of this book, Monte Carlo simulated data will be considered empirical results as if they were measurements. A model that interpolates simulated x-ray spectra will be termed empirical and a model that uses a mix of theoretical and simulated results will be termed semi-empirical. This is reasonable, as, ultimately, such models are agnostic over whether their "empirical" input data come from measurement or simulation.

5.3.1   A closer look at bremsstrahlung

We will distinguish different orders of semi-empirical models, reflecting the mathematical form of the models (but not necessarily the accuracy). Models that can be reduced to a closed-form expression without integrals will be termed zeroth-order models. The Kramers-Whiddington thick-target result is the classic example of a zeroth-order model. Storm also presented zeroth-order models [102] as did Iles [103], the latter probably having the distinction of being the first to present a semi-empirical model making use of Pratt's bremsstrahlung cross sections.

A model involving a single numerical integration over the electron kinetic energy (E) or depth in the target (x) will be termed first-order. Models involving numerical integrations over *both* E and x will be termed second-order. The term third-order will be reserved for models that involve integrals over both E and x, but also the electron direction, $\hat{\Omega}_{\mathrm{e}}$.

Most semi-empirical models of bremsstrahlung spectra can be reduced to the first-order schema [27–30, 102, 104],

$$
\begin{aligned}
\Phi_k^{(1)}(k; Z, E_0) &= \frac{n}{4\pi r^2} H(k) \int_0^{x_{\max}} \frac{\mathrm{d}\sigma_{\mathrm{br}}(k; Z, E)}{\mathrm{d}k} f(x, k; Z)\mathrm{d}x \\
&= \frac{n}{4\pi r^2} H(k) \int_k^{V_e} \frac{\mathrm{d}\sigma_{\mathrm{br}}(k; Z, E)}{\mathrm{d}k} f(x, k; Z)\left(\frac{\mathrm{d}E}{\mathrm{d}x}\right)^{-1} \mathrm{d}E,
\end{aligned}
$$
(5.17)

where Φ_k is the fluence spectrum per incident electron and r is the distance between the source and detection plane. The function $H(k)$ represents an exponential attenuation term arising from inherent and added filtration. The function $f(x, k; Z)$ represents another exponential term defining depth-dependent attenuation of the emissions by the target itself (i.e. self-filtration). The generalized form is,

$$
f(x, k; Z) = \exp\left(-\mu(k; Z)x \cos\gamma \csc\varphi \sec\vartheta\right),
$$
(5.18)

where $\mu(k; Z)$ is the linear attenuation coefficient of the target, φ is the take-off angle, γ is the angle of the electron with respect to the normal to the anode surface (see fig. 2.5a) and ϑ is the out-of-plane angle. Most generally, $\varphi = \alpha + \beta + \delta$, where α is the tube tilt, β is the anode angle and δ is the off-axis angle.

The precise form for the self-filtration term varies between models, as it depends on whether the electron is assumed incident normal to the target ($\gamma = 0$) or normal to the central axis ($\gamma = \beta$). The tube tilt, α, is typically assumed to be zero, as are, often, the off-axis angle, δ, and out-of-plane angle, ϑ. With these conditions, eq. (5.18) simplifies to $f(x, k; Z) = \exp(-\mu(k; Z)x \csc\beta)$ or $f(x, k; Z) = \exp(-\mu(k; Z)x \cot\beta)$, depending on whether electron incidence is assumed normal to the target or not[1].

In some publications, following the notation of Evans [105], the bremsstrahlung cross section is expressed in terms of a scaled quantity, B. This is defined as,

$$
\frac{\mathrm{d}\sigma_{\mathrm{br}}(k; Z, E)}{\mathrm{d}k} = \sigma_0 \frac{E + mc^2}{k\,E} Z^2 B(k; Z, E),
$$
(5.19)

---

[1] When tilt is present or the position required is displaced from the central axis, it can be accounted for in models only accepting an anode angle using the concept of an effective anode angle, such that $\beta_{\mathrm{eff}} = \varphi = \alpha + \beta + \delta$, with either $\gamma = 0$ or $\gamma = \beta_{\mathrm{eff}}$ implied.

where $\sigma_0 = r_e^3 mc/\hbar$. The motivation is the same as for the definition of the scaled cross section χ, introduced in Section 3.2, i.e., the quantities are scaled so that they vary only slowly with E, Z, and k/E.

The bremsstrahlung cross section choice differs between models. Theoretical, theoretically-inspired and entirely empirical parameterizations have been tried. Note that nowhere has the *angle* of bremsstrahlung emission relative to the electron direction been specified. Rather, emissions are expected to be uniformly distributed over 4π radians. This is typically justified by appealing to the fact the electrons quickly reach a diffuse distribution of directions in a thick target, due to multiple-elastic scattering, making the observed distribution insensitive to the intrinsic angular distribution of bremsstrahlung.

In addition to the bremsstrahlung cross section, decisions on electron transport are also key choices. The electron transport, in a first-order model, consists of two aspects. Firstly, for a given tube potential, the relationship between depth and the electron energy, $x(E)$, must be specified. Secondly, the quantity $\mathrm{d}E/\mathrm{d}x$ must be defined. For either decision, the Whiddington (or similar) relation can be used, or a stopping-power formula. While this might just appear to be a choice between simplicity (Whiddington) and accuracy (stopping power), the matter is more complicated. The stopping power is expressed in terms of path length, not penetration depth. Electrons follow tortuous paths in the target and the penetration depth is appreciably less than the total path length. The continuous-slowing-down-approximation (CSDA) range is an average total path-length estimate and derived from the stopping power (see Section 4.1.2). Electrons reach depths in the target up to only approximately half the CSDA range (see fig. 3.2). If correction is not made for this, using a stopping-power formula will over-estimate electron penetration and therefore overestimate the self-filtration of bremsstrahlung by the target.

In 1972, Storm published a seminal article [102]. Given the practical limitations of the Monte Carlo approach, Storm's work can be viewed as an attempt to create a practical analytical model for thick target bremsstrahlung using the best available physics results. First-order and zero-order (referred to as semi-empirical therein) results were presented. Both the Sommerfeld and (Elwert-corrected) Bethe-Heitler bremsstrahlung cross section were trialled in the first-order model. Corrections were made for electron backscatter out of the target as well as for target self-filtration. Stopping power was used to define both the electron energy at depth and $\mathrm{d}E/\mathrm{d}x$ and bremsstrahlung emission was assumed uniform (isotropic). Overall agreement with absolute measurements was quoted as 20% after empirical correction. It was not possible to distinguish whether the Sommerfeld or Bethe-Heitler cross section performed better. Storm concluded that the main weaknesses of the approach were the assumption of isotropic emission and the lack of inclusion of electron path-length detours.

Soole's work, during the period 1972-1976 [27, 106], can be viewed as a pivot away from models which implement the best theoretical results, towards models which work best, in terms of final predictions of beam-quality (e.g.

half-value layer) and, to some extent, tube output (e.g. total fluence or air kerma). His papers were primarily published in medical physics journals, as were those of most of the papers subsequently discussed in this section. In 1976 [27], Soole's work culminated in a semi-empirical model where the theoretical bremsstralung cross section, B, was replaced by a third-order polynomial of k/E, determined empirically by fitting to beam attenuation data. Both the electron energy at depth and dE/dx were defined using the Whiddington relation. No spectra were presented, but Soole was able to accurately reproduce published attenuation curves for tube potentials between 50 and 100 kV.

In 1979, Birch and Marshall built on Soole's contributions [28]. Their model was different in some details. While they defined electron energy at depth using the Whiddington relation, they set dE/dx to be stopping power. They used a fourth-order polynomial of the variable k/E for the product, EB. Notably, they adjusted B based on x-ray spectra measured with a Ge(Li) detector, at a variety of anode angles (10° to 30°), tube voltages (30 to 150 kV), and added filtrations (1 to 4 mm). The article is also clear and straightforward, inviting implementation by others. We note that in adapting Soole's expressions, Birch and Marshall apparently introduced an error into the scaling of the quantity B (by a factor E/mc^2: see eq. (4) in [28]). Since the expression for B was empirically and consistently derived, however, this did not invalidate the work. The model was used for the landmark beam-quality tables published by the Hospital Physics Association in the UK [107]. Later, in 1997, Birch and Marshall's model formed the basis for IPEM Report 78 and the associated software application, distributed on a CD-ROM (including molybdenum and rhodium targets for mammography) [12].

Tucker, Barnes, and Chakraborty revisited Birch and Marshall's approach in 1991 [29]. They corrected the erroneous scaling factor which enabled them to fit B as a fourth-order polynomial in k/E. To accurately describe the output of a tube (in μGy/mAs) they found it necessary to introduce an extra factor, $a + b \, Ve$. From a practical perspective, this was sensible as it enabled the tube output to be successively modelled. The modification does, however, preclude the interpretation of B as a physical quantity. To do so would suggest that the electron at depth "remembers" what its incident energy was. B was fitted to data (70 to 140 kV) more rigorously (in a least-squares sense) than Birch and Marshall's. A model for mammography and a molybdenum target soon followed [104]. The models are available in a free and open-source MATLAB toolkit called xrTk [108].

The work of Blough *et al* [30], published in 1998, deserves mention. A model was presented for mammographic spectra with tungsten, molybdenum, and rhodium targets. While the form of the semi-empirical model was similar to those just discussed, Blough took the notable step of returning to the use of a theoretical bremsstrahlung cross section. The non-relativistic approximation to the Bethe-Heitler formula was used, with an Elwert-type correction for Coulomb effects. Good agreement with half-value-layer measurements was demonstrated for the limited mammography energy range (W:41-47 kV; Mo: 26-29 kV; Rh: 27-30 kV).

These models worked to varying extents and some of them are still used today. However, in reality, electrons do not penetrate in straight lines, they do not have definite predictable energy at a given depth and they do not all penetrate to the same depth. In fact, in tungsten, around 50% of the incident electrons backscatter out again. The authors of the first-order models were not ignorant of these facts. But is begs the question: was an empirical bremsstrahlung cross section typically necessary simply because the model for electron transport in a target was so simplified? And if so, can such models be considered reliable outside the ranges of tube voltages and anode angles they were fitted to? To overcome the limitations, in 2007, Poludniowski [57] extended the semi-empirical form to second-order,

$$
\begin{aligned}
\Phi_k^{(2)}(k; Z, E_0) = d\frac{n}{4\pi r^2} H(k) \int_0^{x_{\max}} \mathrm{d}x \ f(x, k; Z) \\
\times \int_k^E \mathrm{d}E \frac{\mathrm{d}\sigma_{\mathrm{br}}(k; Z, E)}{\mathrm{d}k} \frac{\mathrm{d}N_{\mathrm{pl}}^{\mathrm{e}}(x, E; Z, E_0)}{\mathrm{d}E},
\end{aligned} \tag{5.20}
$$

where $\mathrm{d}N_{\mathrm{pl}}^{\mathrm{e}}(x, E; Z, E_0)/\mathrm{d}E$ is the frequency density of electrons with energy E that pass through a plane at depth, x, per incident electron. The electron frequency density was pre-calculated by Monte Carlo simulation [109]. The constant d (set to 2) is a correction factor for the fact that the path length of an electron is larger than its penetration depth. The Bethe-Heitler cross section was used with a modified interpretation of the Elwert correction, although the NIST tabulations [40] (see Section 3.2.1) were also tested. For more than a decade, the model has been publicly available as a software application called SpekCalc [110], although only a limited version is currently free [111]. The model, with either the Bethe-Heitler and NIST cross sections, is also freely available in the open-source Python toolkit SpekPy by Bujila et al. [1].

The approach embodied by SpekCalc has three principal deficiencies. Firstly, it assumes that the incident electrons instantly achieve a state of diffusion in the target (allowing a constant value for the parameter d). Secondly, an Elwert-corrected Bethe-Heitler bremsstrahlung cross section is used, rather than the more accurate NIST tabulations. Thirdly, it assumes that the distribution of electrons is sufficiently diffuse that the bremsstrahlung emission is uniform (isotropic).

Hernandez and Fernandez [58] began the work of addressing these deficiencies by implementing the NIST cross section and introducing a depth-dependent parameter, $d(x)$. Their model is available in the free and open-source software called xpecgen [112]. Subsequently, the deficiencies of the second-order approach were fully overcome by Omar et al [59, 113], with the introduction of a third-order model. The electron frequency was expressed as a function of electron direction ($\hat{\boldsymbol{\Omega}}_{\mathrm{e}}$) as well as of depth and energy: $N_{E,\hat{\boldsymbol{\Omega}}_{\mathrm{e}}}^{\mathrm{e}}(x, E, \hat{\boldsymbol{\Omega}}_{\mathrm{e}}; Z, E_0)$ (see eq. (6.2) in the next chapter). In addition, the accurate theoretical results of Kissel-Quarles-Pratt (KQP) were used for the bremsstrahlung angular distribution [39]. A full exposition of the approach is provided in Chapter 6. The model agrees closely with measured spectra and Monte Carlo simulations and is available in the SpekPy-v2 toolkit [2].

Table 5.2 summarizes the semi-empirical bremsstrahlung models that have been discussed.

5.3.2 A closer look at characteristic x-rays

The majority of the models discussed in this chapter have been developed for tungsten anode x-ray tubes, where the characteristic emission is assumed to constitute a small contribution to the total output of the tube. The K-line contributions have therefore generally been treated in a cruder approximation than the continuous spectrum and the L-lines have sometimes been neglected entirely.

The L-line contributions (at around 10 keV for tungsten) can indeed be neglected for transmission imaging of humans using x rays, as they are effectively removed by the filtration of the x-ray tube. In other applications, this may not be the case. Notably, Primary Standards Dosimetry Laboratories often include lightly-filtered x-ray beams of low tube potential (<50 kV) in their reference sets for which L-lines can be a substantial contribution. In some applications, such as non-destructive testing with x-ray diffraction (XRD), the characteristic radiation itself is desired [114].

As early as the 1920s, it was known that the fluence of K-line characteristic x-rays from a thin target approximately follows the empirical relation [115],

$$\Phi^{\mathrm{ch}} = C_{\mathrm{K}} \left(E_0 - k_{\mathrm{K}} \right)^{n_{\mathrm{K}}} \tag{5.21}$$

where k_{K} is the K-edge absorption energy and C_{K} and n_{K} are empirical parameters ($1.5 < n_{\mathrm{K}} < 2.0$). This is sometimes referred to as the Webster or Webster-Clark relation. The relation can also be used to model the L-line fluence, if the K-edge energy is replaced with the L-edge energy and different values for the empirical parameters are used. The Webster relation has also been shown to be approximately valid for thick-targets [116], although the observed fluence is dependent on the angle of emission, due to variable target self-filtration. Various suggestions of how to correct the empirical formula for target self-filtration have been made [29, 116].

Theoretical attempts to predict the fluence of characteristic x rays also go back to the first decades of the twentieth century [115, 117, 118]. The problem is complicated by the fact that these emissions are generated by two separate processes: electron impact ionization of the inner shells of the target atoms and atom-photon interactions between bremsstrahlung and the target atoms (see Section 3.3). These two contributions are often referred to as *direct* and *indirect* emissions, in a terminology already in use in the 1920s. Generally, neither contribution can be neglected with respect to the other in thick targets (again, see Section 3.3). However, for the K-shell and

Table 5.2: Summary of semi-empirical bremsstrahlung models. Abbreviations: EBH—Elwert-corrected Bethe-Heitler bremsstrahlung cross section [46, 98]; NIST—NIST bremsstrahlung cross section [40]; KQP—Kissel, Quarles and Pratt bremsstrahlung shape function [39]; W—Whiddington relation [73]; S—stopping power. Under *Bremsstrahlung cross section*: a, b and a_i are fitted coefficients. Under *Geometry conditions*: φ, γ, and ϑ are the take-off, electron, and out-of-plane angle, respectively, entered into eq. (5.18). The effective anode angle is, $\beta_{\text{eff}} = \alpha + \beta + \delta$, where α, β, and δ are the tube tilt, anode angle, and off-axis angle, respectively. For *Electron transport*: e.g. W/S indicates that the Whiddington relation is used to define the electron energy at depth, but the stopping power to define $\mathrm{d}E/\mathrm{d}x$. See the text for the definitions of $\mathrm{d}N_{\text{pl}}^{\text{e}}(x, E; Z, E_0)/\mathrm{d}E$, $d(x)$ and $N_{E,\hat{\Omega}_{\mathbf{e}}}^{\text{e}}(x, E, \hat{\Omega}_{\mathbf{e}}; Z, E_0)$.

Model	Bremsstrahlung cross section ($d\sigma_{\text{br}}/dk$)	Shape function	Geometry conditions	Electron transport
Kramers (1923) [87]	$\frac{16\pi mc}{3\sqrt{3}\hbar} r_{\text{e}}^3 \frac{Z^2}{k\beta^2}$	$\frac{1}{4\pi}$	N/A	W/W
Storm (1972) [102]	Sommerfeld, EBH	$\frac{1}{4\pi}$	$\varphi = \gamma = \beta_{\text{eff}}$ $\vartheta = 0$	S/S
Soole (1976) [27]	$\frac{E+mc^2}{kE}\sum_{i=0}^{3} a_i \left(\frac{k}{E}\right)^i$	$\frac{1}{4\pi}$	$\varphi = \beta_{\text{eff}}$ $\vartheta = 0,\ |\gamma| \geq 0$	W/W
Birch (1979) [28]	$\frac{E+mc^2}{kEmc^2}\sum_{i=0}^{4} a_i \left(\frac{k}{E}\right)^i$	$\frac{1}{4\pi}$	$\varphi = \gamma = \beta_{\text{eff}}$ $\vartheta = 0$	W/S
Tucker (1991) [29]	$\frac{E+mc^2}{kE}(a + b\,Ve)$ $\times \sum_{i=0}^{4} a_i \left(\frac{k}{E}\right)^i$	$\frac{1}{4\pi}$	$\varphi = \beta_{\text{eff}}$ $\gamma = \vartheta = 0$	W/S
Blough (1998) [30]	EBH (non-relativistic)	$\frac{1}{4\pi}$	$\varphi = \beta_{\text{eff}}$ $\gamma = \vartheta = 0$	W/S
Poludniowski (2007) [57]	EBH (modified)	$\frac{1}{4\pi}$	$\varphi = \beta_{\text{eff}}$ $\gamma = \vartheta = 0$	$2\frac{\mathrm{d}N_{\text{pl}}^{\text{e}}}{\mathrm{d}E}$
Fernandez (2016) [58]	NIST	$\frac{1}{4\pi}$	$\varphi = \beta_{\text{eff}}$ $\gamma = 0,\ |\vartheta| \geq 0$	$d(x)\frac{\mathrm{d}N_{\text{pl}}^{\text{e}}}{\mathrm{d}E}$
Bujila (2020) [1]	NIST	$\frac{1}{4\pi}$	$\varphi = \beta_{\text{eff}}$ $\gamma = 0,\ |\vartheta| \geq 0$	$2\frac{\mathrm{d}N_{\text{pl}}^{\text{e}}}{\mathrm{d}E}$
Omar (2021) [59]	NIST	KQP	$\varphi = \beta_{\text{eff}}$ $\gamma = 0,\ |\vartheta| \geq 0$	$N_{E,\hat{\Omega}_{\mathbf{e}}}^{\text{e}}$

high atomic number targets such as tungsten, the indirect contribution is the largest, while the reverse is true for lower atomic number targets such as copper and molybdenum [119]. For the L-shell, the direct component is dominant, even for tungsten [120].

Theoretical approaches to the direct component in thick targets have typically been based on the use of an electron ionization impact cross section in a first-order model. This can be exemplified, for the K-shell, by,

$$\Phi^{\mathrm{dir}(1)}(Z, E_0, k_{\mathrm{K}}) = \frac{n}{4\pi r^2} H(k)\omega_{\mathrm{K}}$$

$$\times \int_k^{Ve} \sigma_{\mathrm{si}}(E; Z, k_{\mathrm{K}}) F(x; Z) \left(\frac{\mathrm{d}E}{\mathrm{d}x}\right)^{-1} \mathrm{d}E, \qquad (5.22)$$

where $\sigma_{\mathrm{si}}(E; Z, k_{\mathrm{K}})$ is the inner shell electron ionization impact cross section, ω_K is the fluorescence yield and $F(x; Z)$ is a function incorporating target self-filtration. Various impact ionization cross sections have been tried, although that due to Mott and Massey is probably the simplest and most widely used [30, 116, 119]. The result is related to the Bethe formula, but with consideration of the ionization of a particular subshell. For the K-shell it can be written as,

$$\sigma_{\mathrm{si}}(E; Z, k_{\mathrm{K}}) = 2\pi r_{\mathrm{e}}^2 m^2 c^4 \frac{1}{Ek_{\mathrm{K}}} b_{\mathrm{K}} \ln\left(\frac{4E}{B_{\mathrm{K}}}\right), \qquad (5.23)$$

where b_{K} and B_{K} are constants. Other impact ionization cross sections such as the relativistic results of Arthurs and Moiseiwitsch [121] and of Kolbenstvedt [122] have also been tried [116] as well as additional corrections for backscatter of incident electrons out of the target.

A typical approach to calculating the indirect component in thick targets presupposes that we know the bremsstrahlung spectrum. Any bremsstrahlung x ray with energy above the subshell edge has the potential to subsequently interact with a target atom and produce a characteristic emission. Given a bremsstrahlung spectrum, it is the task of the model builder to estimate the probability that a bremsstrahlung x ray produces a characteristic x ray, and, ideally, the probability it escapes the target without reabsorption. Webster took this approach in 1927 [123] and several other authors have done so since [57, 116, 119, 124]. We will not attempt to summarize all the model variants. Probably the simplest approach, however, is to assume that half of the bremsstrahlung emissions above the K-edge are reabsorbed. The rationale for this is that bremsstrahlung is produced close to the surface of the target, and that, for isotropic emission, half of these x rays will be oriented into the thick target and absorbed, while the other half have a high probability of escape. The indirect portion of the K-shell characteristic fluence is then,

$$\Phi^{\mathrm{ind}(1)}(Z, E_0, k_{\mathrm{K}}) = \frac{1}{4\pi r^2} H(k)\frac{1}{2} f_{\mathrm{K}}\omega_{\mathrm{K}} \int_{k_{\mathrm{K}}}^{Ve} \Phi_k(k; Z, E_0)\,\mathrm{d}k, \qquad (5.24)$$

where f_K is the fraction of photoelectric absorption that results in a K-shell ionization. For tungsten, f_K is known to take a value of around 0.8 [57,102].

Notably, the expression above does not account for self-filtration of the characteristic emissions by the target. To do so requires an assumption for the depth distribution of characteristic emissions in the target. This can be estimated experimentally [125] or theoretically [123], or even some ansatz can be assumed [29]. In the twenty-first century, a practical and accurate approach is Monte Carlo simulation [120].

Dyson's book [119] and Storm's paper on characteristic emissions from thick targets [116] give excellent summaries of models developed up until the 1970s. More recent implementations, used in thick-target models, are summarized in table 5.3.

Table 5.3: Summary of models of characteristic x-ray emission.

Model	Series	Notes on characteristic emission
Storm (1972) [116]	K,L	Webster's empirical relation ($n_K = 1.67$, $n_L = 1.50$) Eq. (5.21), with no self-filtration
Birch (1979) [28]	K, L	Webster's empirical relation ($n_K = 1.63$, $n_L = 1.63$) Eq. (5.21), with no self-filtration
Tucker (1991) [29]	K	Webster's empirical relation ($n_K = 1.65$) Eq. (5.21), with ansatz depth distribution
Blough (1998) [30]	K	*Direct* contribution only Eq. (5.22), with Mott and Massey cross section
Poludniowski (2007) [57]	K	*Indirect* contribution plus empirical correction Eq. (5.24), multiplied by $(1 + P)$ (P is empirical correction for *direct* emissions)
Fernandez (2016) [58]	K	*Indirect* contribution plus empirical correction Modification of eq. (5.24), with additional polynomial correction
Bujila (2020) [1]	K, L	*Indirect* contribution plus empirical correction Eq. (5.24), with normalization to Monte Carlo simulations that included the *direct* contribution
Omar (2018) [120]	K, L	Monte Carlo simulation of *direct* and *indirect* contributions. The number of emissions and depth distributions were tabulated

5.3.3 Empirical approaches

We have briefly discussed a simple empirical result for bremsstrahlung—see eq. (5.6)—and for characteristic emission—see eq. (5.21). In addition to the theoretical and semi-empirical approaches, it is possible to base the description of the total x-ray spectrum (bremsstrahlung plus characteristic) on entirely empirical data. Arguably, the advantages to do so are that:

- No questionable assumptions about the underlying physics are made (because no assumptions are made regarding particle interactions)

- The empirical model will reproduce measured data accurately, at least for the x-ray tubes and settings used to build the model

Disadvantages are that:

- The empirical model is only as good as the quality of the input data

- Extrapolating to x-ray tubes and settings unlike the input data is problematic

There is no decisive argument in favour of theoretical/semi-empirical or entirely empirical models. A flawed semi-empirical is inferior to a sound empirical model, properly used, and vice versa.

A number of empirical models are in use today. One class of model takes a set of measurements or simulations and interpolates to intermediate settings, for example between tube potentials. In the field of medical physics, Boone has been instrumental in the development of these types of models [126–129]. The TASMIP model (Tungsten Anode Spectral Model using Interpolating Polynomials) was introduced in 1997 for general radiography applications and based on the interpolation of measured spectra between tube voltages [126]. Versions for mammography soon followed, for tungsten ($TASMIP_M$), molybdenum ($MASMIP_M$) and rhodium ($RASMIP_M$) anodes [127]. These models have been widely used. In 2014, a next generation was presented: TASMICS (Tungsten Anode Spectral Model using Interpolating Cubic Splines) [128]. This was based on Monte Carlo simulated spectra, instead of measurements, and, used a different interpolation scheme. The motivations for developing TASMICS included certain deficiencies in the measured data used for TASMIP, the fact that tube design an usage had evolved in the intervening years, and the need for extending the tube potential range. Versions tailored to digital mammmgraphy, breast tomosynthesis, and breast CT systems followed, for tungsten and other anode materials ($TASMICS_{M-T}$, $MASMICS_{M-T}$, $RASMICS_{M-T}$, $TASMICS_{bCT}$) [129]. Both the *ASMIP and *ASMICS families of models are still in use today and a subset of them is available in the Spektr-v3 software [130].

Another class of empirical method is spectrum estimation based on a set of beam attenuation measurements with different thicknesses of material. It asks the question: what spectrum would produce attenuation data like this? This is therefore an inverse problem. There are a variety of ways to reconstruct an estimate of the initial spectrum [131–135]. This empirical approach has a different philosophy to the other models discussed, as it does not produce a generic spectrum for specific settings or design, but provides one tailored to the specific tube. An associated advantage is that it requires no knowledge of the tube design. The measurements necessary are, however, relatively extensive compared to other modelling approaches, which might require none, or simply a half-value layer to tune predictions. An additional challenge is to provide estimates that are robust (not sensitive to small deviations in measurements), particularly for spectra that are not smooth, for example, when characteristic radiation or the effects of absorption edges are present.

5.4 A BRIEF COMPARISON OF MODEL PREDICTIONS

Table 5.4 summarizes software implementing many of the models described in this chapter.

Figure 5.1a shows a tungsten-target bremsstrahlung spectrum predicted from the Kramers-Whiddington model—eq. (5.11)—for a 35 kV tube potential, compared to predictions of two physics models included in the SpekPy-v2 toolkit. All results are normalized to unit fluence. In both SpekPy predictions, the electron transport is treated in the full third-order approach described in the next chapter (our gold standard method). The bremsstrahlung cross sections and angular distributions are treated differently, however, in the two SpekPy results. In the "classical" physics model, Kramers classical cross section—eq. (5.7)—is used, while the angular distribution is assumed uniform. In the "kqp" physics model, the NIST bremsstrahlung cross sections are used, in combination with the Kissel-Quarles-Pratt shape function. It is clear that the Kramers-Whiddington spectra is too soft, as expected, due to the lack of target self-filtration. The classical cross section and uniform emission, however, when combined with accurate electron transport in the target, provides an almost identical result to the quantum mechanical model. This is unsurprising if reference is made to figs. 3.5 and 3.6, where it can be observed that the scaled cross section (χ) and the shape function (S) are relatively flat for the electron energies in question.

The absolute fluence profiles across an x-ray beam (anode-cathode direction) are presented in fig. 5.1b, for the same models. The Kramers-Whiddington model includes no dependence on take-off angle, except that due to distance-squared, producing an almost uniform beam up to the anode grazing angle. The other two models show marked heel effects, with similar behaviour, but quantitative differences.

Figures 5.2a and 5.2b again show the spectra and absolute fluence predictions, this time for a tube potential of 100 kV (with characteristic emissions omitted). As expected, the classical model performs less well at this high potential, where the incident electrons energy must be considered relativistic. It is probably reasonable to conclude, however, that predictions are less sensitive to the precise treatment of the bremsstrahlung cross section and shape functions than the electron transport (i.e., how many electrons reach a certain depth, with specific energy and direction).

Table 5.4: List of x-ray spectrum prediction software. Tube details are specified as: target material (tube potentials, anode angles).

Model	Available software	Tube details
Storm	XPECT v3.5 [136]	W/Mo (1–1000 kV, arbitrary)
Birch	IPEM78 [12]	W (30–150 kV, 6–22°) Mo/Rh (25–32 kV, 9–23°)
Tucker	xrTk [108]	W (10–300 kV, arbitrary) Mo (4–100 kV, arbitrary)
Boone	Spektr-v3 [130] genspec1.c [137] mamspec.c [138]	W (20–150 kV, fixed) W (30–140 kV, fixed) W/Mo/Rh (18-40 kV, fixed)
Poludniowski	SpekCalc [111] SpekPy-v1 [71]	W (30–300 kV, arbitrary) W (15–1000 kV, arbitrary)
Hernandez	TASMICS [128] ∗ASMICS$_{M-T/bCT}$ [129] Spektr-v3 [128]	W (20–640 kV, fixed) W/Mo/Rh$_{M-T}$ (20–49 kV, fixed) W$_{bCT}$ (35–70 kV, fixed) W (20–640 kV, fixed)
Fernandez	xpecgen [112]	W (50–640 kV, arbitrary)
Bujila	SpekPy-v1 [1]	W (15–1000 kV, arbitrary)
Omar	SpekPy-v2 [2]	W (20–300 kV, arbitrary) Mo/Rh (20–50 kV, arbitrary)

Table 5.5 provides a comparison of several analytical models and benchmark Monte Carlo simulations for a variety of beam qualities and tungsten and molybdenum anodes [113]. The first and second half-value layers and the mean mass energy-absorption coefficients in air are presented for TASMICS/MASMICS, IPEM 78, SpekCalc, SpekPy-v1, xpecgen, and SpekPy-v2 (kqp). The results correspond to three different take-off angles (3°, 12° and 21°). Note that for IPEM 78, the closest selectable angle was used. Models that have a fixed take-off angle (TASMICS and MASMICS), perform poorly at very low or high take-off angle. Models not including characteristic

Table 5.5: Relative difference (%) in first and second aluminium half-value layer thickness (HVL$_1$ and HVL$_2$) and the energy-fluence weighted mean value of the mass energy-absorption coefficient in air ($\overline{(\mu_{en}/\rho)_{air}}$) for spectra predicted by various software compared with narrow-beam Monte Carlo calculations using the PENELOPE code system (PEN). Results are presented for a take-off angle (or effective anode angle) of $\varphi = 3°$, $12°$ and $21°$. Data reproduced from ref. [113].

Software	$\varphi = 3°$			$\varphi = 12°$			$\varphi = 21°$		
	HVL$_1$	HVL$_2$	$(\mu_{en}/\rho)_{air}$	HVL$_1$	HVL$_2$	$(\mu_{en}/\rho)_{air}$	HVL$_1$	HVL$_2$	$(\mu_{en}/\rho)_{air}$
Tungsten, NIST M30 (30 kV, 1 mm Be, 0.5 mm Al)									
TASMICS	-5.4	-12.6	10.9	14.5	5.2	-6.8	19.7	10.1	-10.6
IPEM 78	-4.3	-3.4	4.8	1.5	1.7	-0.4	-0.4	-0.9	1.6
SpekCalc	8.8	1.0	-3.7	11.2	3.0	-5.1	11.9	3.8	-5.6
SpekPy-v1	-5.8	-0.6	1.7	4.0	3.6	-3.8	6.0	4.9	-5.0
xpecgen	16.4	7.1	-9.3	17.6	8.8	-10.1	18.2	9.5	-10.6
SpekPy-v2 (kqp)	0.2	-0.1	0.0	0.2	-0.1	0.1	0.1	-0.2	0.3
PEN (mm Al)	0.47	0.71		0.39	0.59		0.37	0.56	
Tungsten, NIST M100 (100 kV, 3 mm Be, 5.25 mm Al)									
TASMICS	-15.0	-10.4	12.7	0.2	-0.3	0.0	4.6	2.6	-3.0
IPEM 78	-0.4	-0.3	0.2	4.5	2.6	-3.1	1.2	0.4	-0.7
SpekCalc	-0.1	0.5	-0.2	-0.1	0.7	-0.4	-0.1	0.8	-0.4
SpekPy-v1	3.1	2.7	-2.5	3.4	3.3	-3.0	3.6	3.6	-3.1
xpecgen	2.2	1.9	-1.8	2.0	1.9	-1.8	1.9	1.9	-1.7
SpekPy-v2 (kqp)	0.2	0.1	-0.2	0.4	0.5	-0.4	0.2	0.3	-0.3
PEN (mm Al)	6.05	7.67		5.13	6.88		4.91	6.70	
Tungsten, NIST M300 (300 kV, 3 mm Be, 4.25 mm Al, 6.5 mm Sn)									
TASMICS	-0.7	-0.7	-0.4	0.2	0.1	0.1	0.5	0.5	0.3
SpekCalc	0.8	0.8	0.4	1.0	1.1	0.5	1.3	1.3	0.7
SpekPy-v1	0.5	0.5	0.3	0.8	0.8	0.4	1.0	1.0	0.5
xpecgen	0.7	0.7	0.4	0.9	0.9	0.4	1.2	1.2	0.6
SpekPy-v2 (kqp)	0.1	0.1	0.0	0.1	0.1	0.0	0.2	0.2	0.1
PEN (mm Al)	21.56	21.65		21.38	21.47		21.30	21.39	
Molybdenum, NIST Mo/Mo25 (25 kV, 1 mm Be, 0.032 mm Mo)									
MASMICS	-6.8	-6.3	6.9	-1.0	-2.5	2.1	-0.2	-2.1	1.6
IPEM 78	-3.8	-3.7	4.3	0.3	-0.9	0.9	-1.1	-1.9	2.1
SpekPy-v2 (kqp)	-0.2	-0.3	0.2	0.0	0.1	-0.2	-0.3	-0.4	0.2
PEN (mm Al)	0.31	0.40		0.30	0.38		0.29	0.38	

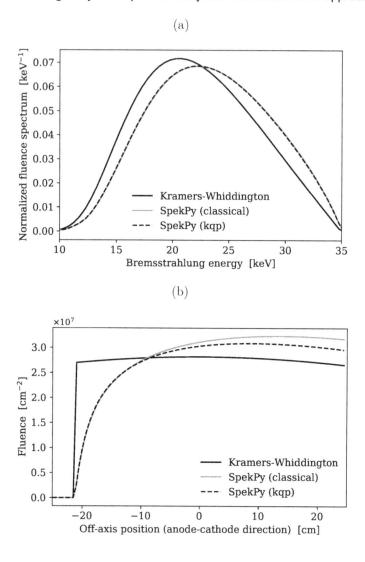

Figure 5.1: (a) Fluence spectra predictions (normalized to unit fluence) for the Kramers-Whiddington, SpekPy-v2 (classical) and SpekPy-v2 (kqp) models, for a tungsten target and 35 kV tube potential. Total filtration is 1 mm of aluminium and the anode angle is 12°. (b) The fluence profile (anode-cathode direction) for the same spectrum, for a 1 mAs exposure at 100 cm source-to-detector distance.

(a)

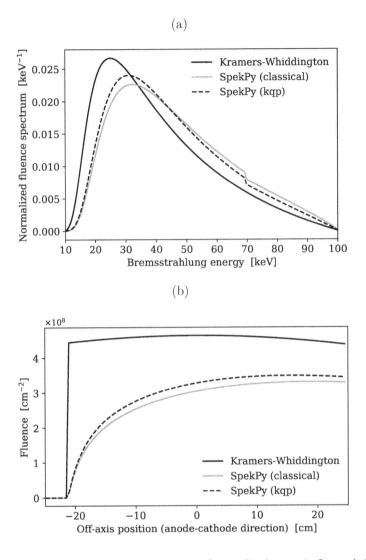

(b)

Figure 5.2: (a) Fluence spectra predictions (normalized to unit fluence) for the Kramers-Whiddington, SpekPy-v2 (classical) and SpekPy-v2 (kqp) models, for a tungsten target and 100 kV tube potential. Total filtration is 1 mm of aluminium and the anode angle is 12°. (b) The fluence profile (anode-cathode direction) for the same spectrum, for a 1 mAs exposure at 100 cm source-to-detector distance.

L-lines, perform poorly for lightly filtered tungsten spectra with low tube potentials (TASMICS, SpekCalc, xpecgen). Away from these predictable cases of failure, all the models produce reasonable predictions for the three metrics, mostly within around 5% of the Monte Carlo predictions.

Table 5.6 provides a comparison of the proportion of characteristic K x rays (α and β lines) to the total, for various models, for an example tungsten spectrum [113]. Measured values are also presented. It can be observed that there is some variation between models, but with only TASMICS and xpecgen showing a substantial departure from measured values.

Table 5.6: Ratio of tungsten K x rays (α and β lines) to the total number of x rays in a spectrum (bremsstrahlung plus characteristic). The spectrum is defined for the central-axis and corresponds to a 100 kV tube potential filtered by 1.2 mm aluminium and 350 cm air. The x-ray target is tungsten and the anode angle 12°. The results are for a variety of software, narrow-beam Monte Carlo calculations (PEN), and measurements. Data reproduced from ref. [113].

Software or data	Method	K_α	K_β	Total
TASMICS	Analytical	0.022	0.006	0.028
IPEM 78	Analytical	0.044	0.012	0.056
SpekCalc	Analytical	0.045	0.013	0.058
SpekPy-v1	Analytical	0.035	0.010	0.045
xpecgen	Analytical	0.017	0.006	0.023
SpekPy-v2 (kqp)	Analytical	0.038	0.011	0.049
PEN	Monte Carlo	0.038	0.011	0.049
Bhat [139]	Measured	0.038	0.011	0.049
Bhat [140]	Measured	0.035	0.012	0.047
Fewell [141]	Measured	0.036	0.010	0.046

5.5   SUMMARY

This chapter summarized a century of developments in analytical models of x-ray tube spectra. It is difficult to be comprehensive, given the span of time and the breadth of applications for x-ray tubes. However, empirical, semi-empirical, and entirely theoretical approaches for predicting x-ray spectra have been discussed. It is natural that the reader might expect some recommendations regarding what models or software to use or avoid. We will refrain from making such recommendations here. All the software presented in the table can be useful, depending on the application and the accuracy required. The user-interface, computer platform, and programming language may also play a role in the reader's choice.

In the next chapter, the model underlying the SpekPy-v2 toolkit will be elaborated in detail, based on the work of Omar *et al.* [51, 59, 113, 120]. The theoretical sophistication is undoubtedly superior to the approaches presented thus far, although whether the improvement in accuracy leads to a decisive practical advantage over other models remains to be seen.

The Python script used for generating figs. 5.1 and 5.2 is available in the repository to this book, at https://bitbucket.org/caxtus. The script is called *classical_approx.py* and uses the SpekPy-v2 toolkit. Try running the script for tube potentials intermediate between 35 and 100 kV. Do you agree with the statement at the end of Section 5.1 that the classical cross section of Kramers loses validity by 50 kV?

CHAPTER 6

An analytical model in detail

A model for x-ray tube spectra is described in this chapter. The model incorporates a detailed treatment of the electron transport, the resulting bremsstrahlung emission, and the production of x rays with characteristic energy. This model has been implemented in the SpekPy-v2 toolkit [2] along with alternative physics models and approximations.

6.1 MODELLING THE EMISSION SPECTRUM

The x-ray spectrum, that is, fluence differential in photon energy k per incident electron with kinetic energy E_0, can be expressed in a general form as,

$$\Phi_k(k, \boldsymbol{r}; Z, E_0) = \Phi_k^{\mathrm{br}} + \Phi_k^{\mathrm{ch}} = G(\boldsymbol{r}) H(k, \hat{\boldsymbol{\Omega}}_\gamma) \left((N_{k,\hat{\boldsymbol{\Omega}}_\gamma}^{\mathrm{br}} + N_{k,\hat{\boldsymbol{\Omega}}_\gamma}^{\mathrm{ch}})(k, \hat{\boldsymbol{\Omega}}_\gamma; Z, E_0) \right),$$

(6.1)

where $N_{k,\hat{\boldsymbol{\Omega}}_\gamma}^{\mathrm{br}}$ and $N_{k,\hat{\boldsymbol{\Omega}}_\gamma}^{\mathrm{ch}}$ are, respectively, the number of bremsstrahlung and characteristic x rays emerging from a target (i.e., the tube anode) of atomic number Z, differential in photon energy k and emission direction $\hat{\boldsymbol{\Omega}}_\gamma$. The conversion to fluence at a point $\boldsymbol{r}$ in the x-ray field and the attenuation of filters is taken into account, respectively, by,

$$G(\boldsymbol{r}) = \|\boldsymbol{r}\|^{-2}. \quad H(k, \hat{\boldsymbol{\Omega}}_\gamma) = \exp\left(-\sum_i \mu_i(k)\, t_i(\hat{\boldsymbol{\Omega}}_\gamma) \right), \qquad (6.2)$$

where $t_i(\hat{\boldsymbol{\Omega}}_\gamma)$ is the thickness of a filter material i in the emission direction $\hat{\boldsymbol{\Omega}}_\gamma$, and μ_i is its linear attenuation coefficient.

Equation (6.1) can be evaluated using an analytic model for the production and filtration of x rays in the target. Such a model was developed from theoretical principles in ref. [142], and is outlined below.

DOI: 10.1201/9781003058168-6

6.1.1 Bremsstrahlung production

Consider the emission of a photon with energy k in direction $\hat{\boldsymbol{\Omega}}_\gamma$ following the deceleration of an electron with kinetic energy E traveling in direction $\hat{\boldsymbol{\Omega}}_e$ in the atomic Coulomb field (geometry illustrated in fig. 6.1). Using these notations, the number of bremsstrahlung photons emerging from an isotropic medium with atomic number Z and atomic density n per incident electron with kinetic energy E_0, can be expressed as,

$$N^{br}_{k,\hat{\boldsymbol{\Omega}}_\gamma}(k,\hat{\boldsymbol{\Omega}}_\gamma;Z,E_0) = n \int_0^\infty dx \int_k^{E_0} dE \int d\hat{\boldsymbol{\Omega}}_e \, N^e_{E,\hat{\boldsymbol{\Omega}}_e}(x,E,\hat{\boldsymbol{\Omega}}_e;Z,E_0)$$

$$\times \frac{d^2\sigma_{br}(k,\hat{\boldsymbol{\Omega}}_e \cdot \hat{\boldsymbol{\Omega}}_\gamma;Z,E)}{dk \, d\hat{\boldsymbol{\Omega}}_\gamma} f_{br}(x,k,\hat{\boldsymbol{\Omega}}_\gamma;Z), \quad (6.3)$$

where $d^2\sigma_{br}/dk d\hat{\boldsymbol{\Omega}}_\gamma$ is the bremsstrahlung cross section double differential in the energy and direction of the emitted photon, and $N^e_{E,\hat{\boldsymbol{\Omega}}_e}(x,E,\hat{\boldsymbol{\Omega}}_e;Z,E_0)$ describes the electron penetration in terms of the number of electrons at depth x in the target per incident electron with energy E_0, differential in kinetic energy E and direction $\hat{\boldsymbol{\Omega}}_e$.

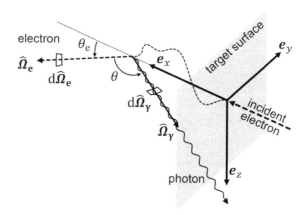

Figure 6.1: Geometry of the bremsstrahlung process. An electron propagating along a unit vector direction $\hat{\boldsymbol{\Omega}}_e$ within the target emits a photon of energy k in direction $\hat{\boldsymbol{\Omega}}_\gamma$. The electron direction is specified by the polar angle θ_e relative to the incidence direction, e_x. The photon emission direction is specified by the polar angle between the direction of the emitted photon and the initial electron direction, $\cos\theta = \hat{\boldsymbol{\Omega}}_e \cdot \hat{\boldsymbol{\Omega}}_\gamma$.

The filtration of bremsstrahlung by overlying target material is accounted for by $f_{br}(x, k, \hat{\boldsymbol{\Omega}}_\gamma; Z)$, which is the transmission of photons with energy k emitted in direction $\hat{\boldsymbol{\Omega}}_\gamma$ from a depth x. This filtration can be determined from the target material's linear attenuation coefficient, μ, as,

$$f_{br}(x, k, \hat{\boldsymbol{\Omega}}_\gamma; Z) = \exp\left(-\mu(k; Z)\, x \csc\varphi \sec\vartheta\right), \qquad (6.4)$$

where φ is the take-off angle defined by $\csc\varphi = \|\boldsymbol{r}_x + \boldsymbol{r}_z\| / \|\boldsymbol{r}_x\|$ in fig. 6.2 and ϑ is the corresponding out-of-plane angle defined by $\sec\vartheta = \|\boldsymbol{r}\| / \|\boldsymbol{r}_x + \boldsymbol{r}_z\|$ (not shown in the figure), given that $\|\boldsymbol{r}\| \gg x$. The above equation can be derived from the generalized expression for the self-filtration that was presented in eq. (5.18), given that $\gamma = 0$, which is to say that the incident electrons are assumed to enter the anode normally. Recall from Chapter 3 that this assumption is supported by the fact that the electric field lines in the inter-electrode space of the x-ray tube end up perpendicular to the surface of the conducting anode.

The electron penetration data entering the model can be determined by Monte Carlo calculation of the number of electrons with kinetic energy E crossing a plane at depth x in the direction $\hat{\boldsymbol{\Omega}}_e$, per incident electron with energy E_0,

$$N^e_{E, \hat{\boldsymbol{\Omega}}_e}(x, E, \hat{\boldsymbol{\Omega}}_e; Z, E_0) = \frac{d^2 N^e_{pl}(x, E, \hat{\boldsymbol{\Omega}}_e; Z, E_0)}{\left|\hat{\boldsymbol{\Omega}}_e \cdot \boldsymbol{e}_x\right| dE \, d\hat{\boldsymbol{\Omega}}_e}, \qquad (6.5)$$

where $\left|\hat{\boldsymbol{\Omega}}_e \cdot \boldsymbol{e}_x\right| = |\cos\theta_e|$ relates the number of electrons at depth x to the number of electrons crossing a plane at that depth, similar to how fluence and planar fluence are related according to eq. (4.2).

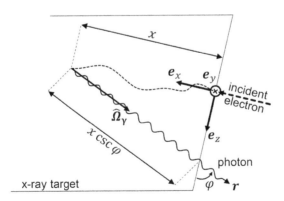

Figure 6.2: Geometry for the emission of bremsstrahlung from a target (i.e., an x-ray tube anode). A photon is emitted in direction $\hat{\boldsymbol{\Omega}}_\gamma$ following a bremsstrahlung interaction at depth x in the target. The emitted photon exits the target with a take-off angle φ as it propagates toward a point $\boldsymbol{r}$.

For efficient numerical integrations, it is convenient to introduce the following decomposition,

$$N^{\mathrm{e}}_{E,\hat{\boldsymbol{\Omega}}_{\mathrm{e}}}(x, E, \hat{\boldsymbol{\Omega}}_{\mathrm{e}}; Z, E_0) = N^{\mathrm{e}}_E(x, E; Z, E_0)\, p_{\hat{\boldsymbol{\Omega}}_{\mathrm{e}}}(\hat{\boldsymbol{\Omega}}_{\mathrm{e}} \mid x, E; Z, E_0), \qquad (6.6)$$

where $N^{\mathrm{e}}_E(x, E)$ is the number of electrons at depth x differential in kinetic energy E,

$$N^{\mathrm{e}}_E(x, E; Z, E_0) = \int d\hat{\boldsymbol{\Omega}}_{\mathrm{e}} \frac{d^2 N^{\mathrm{e}}_{\mathrm{pl}}(x, E, \hat{\boldsymbol{\Omega}}_{\mathrm{e}}; Z, E_0)}{\left|\hat{\boldsymbol{\Omega}}_{\mathrm{e}} \cdot \boldsymbol{e}_x\right| dE\, d\hat{\boldsymbol{\Omega}}_{\mathrm{e}}}, \qquad (6.7)$$

and where $p_{\hat{\boldsymbol{\Omega}}_{\mathrm{e}}}(\hat{\boldsymbol{\Omega}}_{\mathrm{e}} \mid x, E)$ is the conditional probability distribution of the propagation direction of electrons with kinetic energy E at depth x, which can be evaluated as,

$$p_{\hat{\boldsymbol{\Omega}}_{\mathrm{e}}}(\hat{\boldsymbol{\Omega}}_{\mathrm{e}} \mid x, E; Z, E_0) = \frac{d^2 N^{\mathrm{e}}_{\mathrm{pl}}(x, E, \hat{\boldsymbol{\Omega}}_{\mathrm{e}}; Z, E_0)}{\left|\hat{\boldsymbol{\Omega}}_{\mathrm{e}} \cdot \boldsymbol{e}_x\right| dE\, d\hat{\boldsymbol{\Omega}}_{\mathrm{e}}}$$
$$\times \left(\int d\hat{\boldsymbol{\Omega}}_{\mathrm{e}} \frac{d^2 N^{\mathrm{e}}_{\mathrm{pl}}(x, E, \hat{\boldsymbol{\Omega}}_{\mathrm{e}}; Z, E_0)}{\left|\hat{\boldsymbol{\Omega}}_{\mathrm{e}} \cdot \boldsymbol{e}_x\right| dE\, d\hat{\boldsymbol{\Omega}}_{\mathrm{e}}}\right)^{-1}. \qquad (6.8)$$

This decomposition is useful for analyzing certain aspects of the model, such as the energy and depth distribution of bremsstrahlung produced in the x-ray target. These two components of the bremsstrahlung production can be determined from eq. (6.3), as,

$$N^{\mathrm{br}}_k(x, k; Z, E_0) = n \int_k^{E_0} dE\, N^{\mathrm{e}}_E(x, E; Z, E_0)\, \frac{Z^2}{\beta_{\mathrm{i}}^2}\frac{1}{k}\chi(k; Z, E), \qquad (6.9)$$

and

$$N^{\mathrm{br}}(x; Z, E_0) = \int_{k_{\mathrm{cut}}}^{E_0} dk\, N^{\mathrm{br}}_k(x, k; Z, E_0), \qquad (6.10)$$

where β_{i} is the initial electron velocity in units of the speed of light in vacuum, and χ is the scaled energy-weighted bremsstrahlung cross section differential in photon energy (defined in eq. (3.2)). Note that a low-energy cut-off, k_{cut}, is introduced because the expression diverges at $k = 0$.

Numerical evaluations of eqs. (6.9) and (6.10) are presented in figs. 6.3 and 6.4. The calculations were performed using NIST bremsstrahlung cross sections differential in energy (described in Section 3.2.1) combined with pre-calculated Monte Carlo data for the electron penetration extracted from ref. [143]. The results are compared with a full Monte Carlo treatment of the electron-photon transport in the target. Notice the excellent agreement achieved by implementing the same cross sections in the model as used in the Monte Carlo simulations.

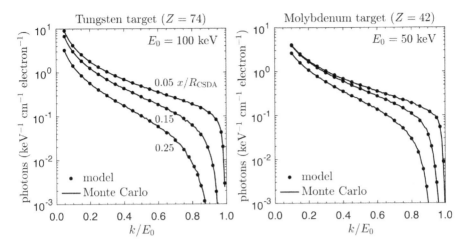

Figure 6.3: Energy spectra of bremsstrahlung produced in a target per incident electron with kinetic energy E_0. The energy is scaled by the incident electron energy (k/E_0). Monte Carlo calculations (PENELOPE [35]) are compared with model results obtained by evaluating eq. (6.9) down to 5 keV photon energy, with NIST bremsstrahlung cross sections and electron penetration data from ref. [143].

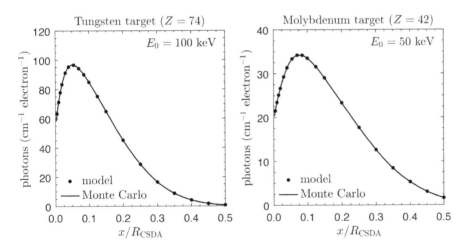

Figure 6.4: Depth distributions of bremsstrahlung produced in a target per incident electron with kinetic energy E_0. The depth is scaled by the CSDA range ($x/R_{\mathrm{CSDA}}(E_0)$). Monte Carlo calculations (PENELOPE [35]) are compared with model results obtained by evaluating eq. (6.10) down to 5 keV photon energy, with NIST bremsstrahlung cross sections and electron penetration data from ref. [143].

According to the above results, the model is able to predict the depth and energy distribution of bremsstrahlung produced in an x-ray target. However, in order to predict the x-ray energy leaving the target in a given direction, the angular distribution of the bremsstrahlung production must also be considered. This can be achieved by accounting for the intrinsic bremsstrahlung angular distribution, i.e., the shape function, given that the directional distribution of the electrons penetrating the target is known.

Previous models have typically assumed, albeit sometimes implicitly, that the intrinsic bremsstrahlung angular distribution is spherically uniform. The rationale has been that electrons emitted from the cathode instantly attain a diffuse directional distribution when they penetrate into the anode. This assumption leads to an overestimation of the number of x rays produced near the target surface, which in turn leads to an overestimation of the x-ray fluence emitted from the target [59]. We can observe this effect in fig. 6.5, which shows model predictions of bremsstrahlung emission from thick tungsten and molybdenum targets. The performance of the present model (implemented according to eq. (6.3)) is compared with model results obtained assuming instant diffusion combined with a uniform intrinsic bremsstrahlung angular distribution (implemented equivalent to eq. (5.20)).

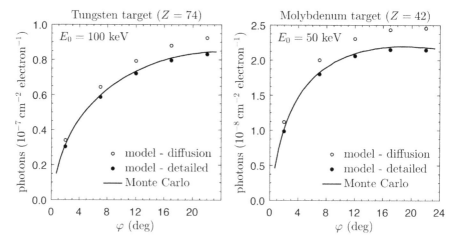

Figure 6.5: Bremsstrahlung fluence calculated for a minimally filtered (1 mm Be and 100 cm air) x-ray tube as a function of the take-off angle, φ, per incident electron with kinetic energy E_0. The results correspond to the model outlined in this chapter (model—detailed) expressed by eq. (6.3) (with the KQP shape function, eq. (3.7)), and previous work assuming instant electron diffusion (model—diffusion) expressed by eq. (5.20) (with uniform shape function). Both models implement electron penetration data from ref. [143], and NIST bremsstrahlung cross sections. Monte Carlo-calculated results (PENELOPE [35]) are included as benchmark.

As expected, the figure demonstrates that assuming instant diffusion combined with a uniform intrinsic bremsstrahlung angular distribution (the shape function) leads to a considerable overestimation (>10%) of the amount of bremsstrahlung emitted from an x-ray tube anode. Implementing a more detailed treatment of the angular distribution of both the electrons penetrating the target as well as the bremsstrahlung shape function, produces results in better agreement with Monte Carlo simulations. It is worth noting that although the model agrees with Monte Carlo to within about 2%, it tends to slightly underestimate the amount of bremsstrahlung emitted. This difference can to some extent be explained by the fact that the model does not consider secondary scatter contributions, that is, all scatterings in the x-ray tube geometry (including the target) are assumed to attenuate the emitted x-ray beam. In reality, and especially for broad x-ray beams, some scattered x rays are deflected toward the region of interest, adding to the x-ray fluence observed. A more in-depth analysis of the influence of scattering is provided in ref. [120], albeit for characteristic x rays.

It should be noted that by factorizing the double differential cross section according to eq. (3.1), the model presented in this chapter can be implemented using different combinations of cross sections for the intrinsic bremsstrahlung energy and angular distribution. Several options for these cross sections were outlined and discussed in Chapter 3.

6.1.2 Characteristic x-ray production

Recall from the theory outlined in Section 3.3 that a photon with characteristic energy is emitted when an atom with a vacancy in one of its inner shells relaxes from its excited state through a radiative transition, that is, by fluorescence. Specific radiative transitions are conveniently described in terms of the atomic shells involved, such as a radiative S0–S1 transition which occurs when a vacancy in an inner-shell S0 is filled by an electron from an outer subshell S1. The energy released in such a transition is correspondingly expressed as k_{S0-S1}. Using these notations, along with those presented in fig. 6.6, the differential number of x rays emerging from a target with a discrete energy k (expressed by the Dirac delta distribution, δ), can be formulated as,

$$N^{ch}_{k,\hat{\Omega}_\gamma}(k, \hat{\Omega}_\gamma; Z, E_0) = \sum_{S0,S1} \delta(k - k_{S0-S1})\, \upsilon_{S0-S1}(Z)$$

$$\times \frac{1}{R_{CSDA}} \int_0^\infty \frac{dx}{4\pi}\, \phi_{S0}(x/R_{CSDA}; Z, E_0)\, f_{ch}(x, k, \hat{\Omega}_\gamma; Z),$$

$$(6.11)$$

where the summation is over all relevant S0–S1 radiative transitions, and ϕ_{S0} is the x-ray fluorescence produced by a vacancy in the inner-shell S0, differential in penetration depth scaled by the electron CSDA range, x/R_{CSDA}, per electron with kinetic energy E_0 incident upon a target of atomic number Z. Furthermore, recall from eq. (3.13) that υ_{S0-S1} is the average number of

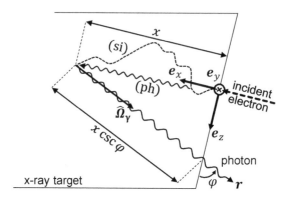

Figure 6.6: Geometry for the emission of characteristic x rays from a target (i.e., an x-ray tube anode). A photon is emitted in direction $\hat{\mathbf{\Omega}}_\gamma$ following inner-shell ionization caused either by electron impact or photon interaction at depth x (illustrated by the two paths labeled (si) and (ph), respectively). The emitted photon exits the target with a take-off angle φ as it propagates toward a point $\mathbf{r}$.

x rays emitted for a given radiative S0–S1 transition per one fluorescence in the target, which can be determined using available tabulations of transition probabilities [63] (relevant data for tungsten shown in fig. 3.9). Note that depth distributions of x-ray fluorescence can be determined using the Monte Carlo method. Such data is available from ref. [60], addressing various x-ray target materials (results for tungsten and molybdenum shown in figs. 3.7 and 3.8).

The filtration of x rays by overlying target material is in eq. (6.11) accounted for by $f_{ch}(x, k, \hat{\mathbf{\Omega}}_\gamma; Z)$, which is the transmission of photons with energy k emitted in direction $\hat{\mathbf{\Omega}}_\gamma$ from a depth x,

$$f_{ch}(x, k, \hat{\mathbf{\Omega}}_\gamma; Z) = \exp\left(-\mu_{wo/co}(k; Z)\, x \csc \varphi \sec \vartheta\right). \tag{6.12}$$

This expression parallels eq. (6.4) for the filtration of bremsstrahlung, except for the important difference that Rayleigh (coherent) scattering is excluded from the linear attenuation coefficient, $\mu_{wo/co}$. The exclusion of Rayleigh scattering is based on the assumption that characteristic radiation is emitted isotropically in a target with randomly oriented atoms. In such case, the angular deflections resulting from Rayleigh interactions have no effect on the number of x rays emerging from the target in a given direction, as the intrinsic Rayleigh scattering angular distribution is masked by the initial isotropic angular distribution. This is to say that the x rays are not attenuated by the process of Rayleigh scattering. This argument cannot be applied to Compton scattering, as in such scattering events energy is lost. Note that, even for Rayleigh scattering, the approximation is imperfect. The initial isotropic angular distribution is expected to become somewhat skewed due to x-ray absorption in the target. Nevertheless, excluding Rayleigh scattering from the linear attenuation coefficient was shown in ref. [120] to be a reasonable first-order approximation that can improve the accuracy of the model by up to 6%.

6.2 IMPLEMENTING THE MODEL

An example implementation of the complete model (bremsstrahlung and characteristic x rays) is demonstrated in this section. The bremsstrahlung spectrum has been implemented as described in Section 6.1.1, using Monte Carlo-calculated electron penetration data from ref. [143], combined with NIST bremsstrahlung cross sections (described in Section 3.2.1) and the parametrized form of the bremsstrahlung shape function by Acosta *et al.* [52] (see eq. (3.7)). The characteristic x-ray emission has been implemented as described in Section 6.1.2, using Monte Carlo-calculated fluorescence depth distributions from ref. [60] combined with transition probabilities from the Livermore EADL database [63] and emission energies compiled by Deslattes *et al.* [144].

Spectra calculated for minimally filtered x-ray tubes are presented in figs. 6.7 and 6.8. The figures show that the model is able to reproduce comprehensive Monte Carlo simulations, with the first and second aluminium half-value layer thicknesses agreeing to within 1%, and the mean spectral energy within 0.5%

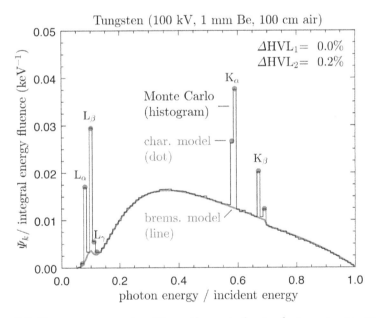

Figure 6.7: X-ray energy spectra, Ψ_k, on the central axis of a tungsten target tilted 12°. The model outlined in this chapter (line and dot) is compared with Monte Carlo simulations (histogram) performed using the PENELOPE code system [35]. Also shown is the relative difference (%) in first and second aluminium half-value layer thickness (ΔHVL).

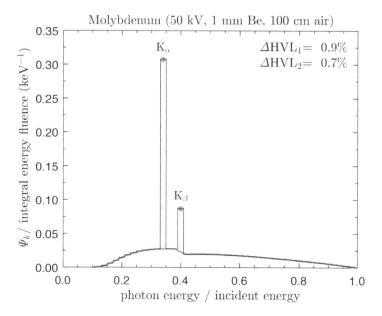

Figure 6.8: X-ray energy spectra, Ψ_k, on the central axis of a molybdenum target tilted $12°$. The model outlined in this chapter (line and dot) is compared with Monte Carlo simulations (histogram) performed using the PENELOPE code system [35]. Also shown is the relative difference (%) in first and second aluminium half-value layer thickness (ΔHVL).

The performance of the model can further be validated by comparing with empirical results, such as the pulse height spectra measured by Ankerhold [20] at PTB, the German Primary Standards Dosimetry Laboratory, using a high-purity Germanium (Ge) detector. The spectra measured for selected IEC RQR/RQA (tungsten) diagnostic beam qualities [145] using a narrow-beam geometry are presented in fig. 6.9, along with the corresponding spectra calculated using the model presented in this chapter. The figure indicates a good agreement in both the continuous bremsstrahlung component and the discrete characteristic x-ray peaks. These results are consistent with the comprehensive evaluation provided in ref. [113], which includes Monte Carlo simulations, measured spectra, and various analytical models. It is also emphasized that a quantitative comparison of model predictions and measured half-value layer thicknesses (HVL) is provided in Chapter 8 for typical x-ray beam qualities available at several Primary Standards Dosimetry Laboratories.

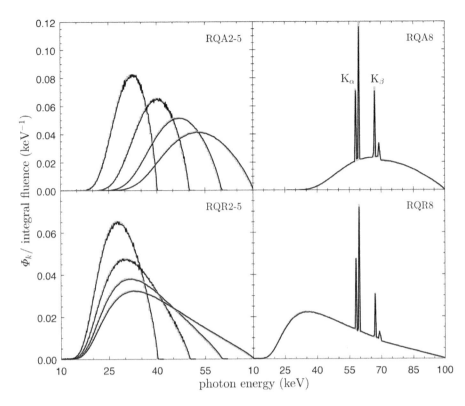

Figure 6.9: X-ray fluence spectra, Φ_k, calculated analytically using the model outlined in this chapter (histogram) and measured by Ankerhold [20] (line) at the German Primary Standards Dosimetry Laboratory (Physikalisch-Technische Bundesanstalt, PTB). The results correspond to selected IEC RQR/RQA (tungsten) diagnostic beam qualities [145] (specified in table 8.1).

A supplementary Python script to this chapter is available in the book's online software repository, at https://bitbucket.org/caxtus. It is called *physics_models.py* and uses the SpekPy-v2 toolkit. The script plots the RQR5 spectrum for four physics models and calculates the first half-value layers. The physics models are (in order of increasing accuracy): "diff", "uni", "sim" and "kqp". Are the differences between fluence spectra consistent with the discussion at the end of Section 6.1.1? Compare the half-value layers. Do you think the full KQP shape function is necessary?

Note on physics models:
"diff"—instant electron diffusion and uniform shape function
"uni"—detailed electron angular distribution and uniform shape function
"sim"—detailed electron angular distribution and SIM shape function
"kqp"—detailed electron angular distribution and KQP shape function

CHAPTER 7

Overview on Monte Carlo modelling

T HE Monte Carlo method is a numerical technique that makes use of repeated random sampling to simulate the behaviour of a complex system. This chapter provides an overview of the general principles of Monte Carlo modelling of x-ray tube spectra and includes a summary of the theory and practical aspects of several widely-used computer code systems that are suitable for this task.

7.1   GENERAL PRINCIPLES

"The question was what are the chances that a Canfield solitaire laid out with 52 cards will come out successfully? After spending a lot of time trying to estimate them by pure combinatorial calculations, I wondered whether a more practical method than 'abstract thinking' might not be to lay it out say one hundred times and simply observe and count the number of successful plays. This was already possible to envisage with the beginning of the new era of fast computers, and I immediately thought of problems of neutron diffusion... " —Stanislaw Ulam

The insight quoted above [146] occurred to the Polish mathematician in 1946, as he passed time by playing cards alone. The principles underlying his idea were not new, but the application to modelling the transport of radiation was, as was the moniker Ulam and his colleagues at Los Alamos came up with to describe the approach: the Monte Carlo method. A comprehensive introduction to the technique will not be given here—there are other excellent texts for that [65, 147]. However, for the sake of the uninitiated, we will give an overview of some critical concepts and terminology.

Just as a game of solitaire consists of a sequence of draws of random cards, the fate of a single initial particle can be described by a sequence of random

DOI: 10.1201/9781003058168-7

events, up to the moment it stops (ending the game). In the jargon of Monte Carlo transport, this is a *particle history*. The distance to the next interaction can be sampled randomly, based on the total cross section of the interaction process. The outcomes of the event, e.g. energy loss and scattering angle, can be sampled from distributions defined by the differential cross sections (i.e. the cross section differential in the quantity being sampled).

The transport of particles such as electrons and photons is, at its most general, a *coupled* transport problem. For example, one particle, such as an x ray, can liberate electrons from atoms, which may in turn, radiate x rays, etc. In principle, all the consequences stemming from that initial particle should be traced, including the stack of secondary particles, before the history can be considered complete. Rules need to be defined for when the game finishes. For a particle, this occurs when it is absorbed, leaves the geometry, or when its energy (or mean free path) falls below a *transport cut-off* and it is then assumed stopped.

Electrons (and other charged particles) pose particular problems for simulation. An energetic electron may scatter elastically many millions of times before it is stopped. To follow each electron's complete *analogue history* is computationally expensive. *Condensed history* techniques have been developed to reduce electron transport into a sequence of steps, with each step bundling the net effect of many interactions. There are many algorithms for doing so, but Berger defined two main types [148]. *Class I* algorithms involve the grouping of all collisions into predetermined steps. *Class II* algorithms, instead, group only *soft* interactions, involving small energy losses and deflections (based on some threshold for small), while sampling *hard* interactions using appropriate single-scattering cross sections. One of the Monte Carlo codes discussed in detail in this chapter employs a Class I scheme, while the others use Class II schemes, although some provide the possibility for full analogue treatment.

The question arises as to how we sample randomly. This can be performed using sequences of numbers sampled on a fixed interval e.g. between 0 and 1. It is possible to use sequences of truly random numbers (e.g. generated by a roulette wheel), but it is more practical to use *pseudo-random number* generators [149]. These are algorithms that generate deterministic sequences that appear random. By starting two identical simulations with different random number *seeds*, two statistically independent simulations can be ensured. In contrast, using the same seeds will produce identical result, which is useful for validating code and correct installation, as well as debugging.

Scoring and *geometry* are linked. To make meaningful simulations, various regions must be represented in code, along with the materials' characteristics and physical extension. There are various ways to do this, including combinations of *planes* and *quadric surfaces* (e.g. ellipsoid, cones, and cylinders), regular matrices (i.e. *voxels*) or other *meshes*. The scoring of statistics is usually based on geometry. Examples are the energy deposited in a region, or the fluence passing through a specified surface. The statistics are often referred to as *tallies*, as the estimates are, in principle at least, updated history-by-history as more particles are simulated. It is also possible to trigger the logging of the spatial and kinematic properties of each particle that passes through a surface. The resulting electronic file is referred to as a *phase-space file*. Advantageously, other information can be scored or logged that can be difficult or impossible to infer experimentally, for example, whether a photon was generated by bremsstrahlung or atomic relaxations, or whether it scattered in a specified region.

There is an *uncertainty* in any tally being scored and the *variance* decreases inversely with the number of histories (due to the Central Limit Theorem of statistics). This means that simulation time must be increased by a factor of 4 to reduce the uncertainty (i.e. the square root of variance) in a tally by a factor of 2. Fortunately, because each history is considered statistically independent, problems are "embarrassingly parallel" and amenable to running in batches on multiple computer cores.

There are other ways to obtain a target uncertainty more quickly. *Variance reduction techniques* are tricks to increase the efficiency of calculations while *speed-up techniques* are approximations that achieve the same goal. One example, for charged particles, is *range rejection*, in which the electrons that cannot feasibly reach a scoring region of interest are stopped immediately, to save the time that would have been wasted on their simulation. There are numerous variance reduction/speed-up techniques and many codes employ some. They must be used with care, because if used incorrectly they may not decrease (and even increase) the simulation time required for a given uncertainty. Speed-up techniques can also introduce *bias* (i.e. systematic shifts) in the predictions.

The reader should appreciate by this point, that setting up simulations for a Monte Carlo system that models coupled electron-photon transport is complex and typically involves many specifications from the user. Figure 7.1 illustrates several of the aspects touched upon above. Despite its challenges, Monte Carlo simulation has become a standard tool in radiation physics for solving radiation transport problems. In the field of medical physics alone, it is used for such diverse applications as estimating patient dose, improving x-ray image reconstructions, optimizing radiotherapy applications, and calculating radiation protection quantities [65, 150–153].

7.2 ASPECTS RELEVANT FOR MODELLING X-RAY TUBES

Monte Carlo systems differ not only in how the Monte Carlo method is implemented but also in the physics models and interaction cross sections applied. Using different Monte Carlo systems can therefore produce slightly (or sometimes even considerably) different results, which is why it is important for the user to be familiar with the approximations and limitations of a particular code. To be used for modelling x-ray tubes, it is essential that a code can simulate both electrons and photons in the kinetic energy range of

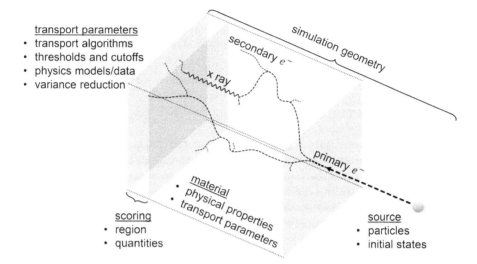

Figure 7.1: Components of a typical coupled electron-photon Monte Carlo simulation. The geometry includes a particle source, scoring region, and geometrical objects with well-defined material properties. The simulation is configured by specifying various global and local (a specific material or region) transport parameters, such as energy transfer thresholds, cut-off energies, variance reduction techniques, transport algorithms, and physics models/data.

around 1 keV to 1000 keV. Further, it must be possible to construct suitable geometries and derive an output spectra, by, for example, scoring fluence through a surface or saving a phase-space file for later analysis.

The sophistication of the simulation geometry depends largely on the physical effect one wishes to study. Take for instance the study of extra-focal radiation from an x-ray tube. In order to study this radiation component produced by backscattered electrons reentering the anode, the inter-electrode vacuum space must be modelled. The transport of electrons in the static electric field between the electrodes should then be simulated using a suitable code system that incorporates the relevant electromagnetic fields transport physics [31, 154]. Another example is the simulation of x-ray tubes with small beam collimators ($\lesssim$ 10 mm diameter aperture) used for precision irradiation of small animals. Such simulations require a realistic model of the focal spot intensity distribution, as the collimators may partially block the focal source (i.e., the finite-sized primary photon source) [154, 155]. Other aspects of the geometry that may be relevant for specialized studies are the surface roughness of the anode [156] and a complete geometrical representation of the x-ray tube housing assembly [157].

Such detailed x-ray tube simulations are useful for the study of a particular radiation effect or tube design. There are, however, various applications for which a simplified geometry is beneficial [113, 128, 158, 159]. The essential components of the geometry are a thick angled slab (the x-ray target), an electron pencil beam (electron source), and slabs placed in the x-ray beam (the x-ray tube filters). An example of such a geometry is illustrated in fig. 2.5 (Section 2.4.2).

Some specific recommendations regarding the Monte Carlo simulation of x-ray production and transport are as follows:

- Modern tabulations of the bremsstrahlung cross section differential in energy should be used (e.g. NIST, NRC, EEDL). Older analytic results, such as that of Bethe-Heitler (see Chapter 5.2.2), should be avoided

- The Kissel-Quarles-Pratt (KQP) shape function for the angular distribution of bremsstrahlung is preferred (see Section 3.2.2), although 2BN and similar (e.g. KM and SIM [34]) are reasonable. Highly relativistic results such as 2BS are not recommended but will not necessarily lead to large discrepancies

- The code should include atomic relaxations due to photon interactions and electron impact ionization (preferably L as well as K shell). The sophistication required in relaxation models, however, depends on the situation being simulated

- The code should include coherent (Rayleigh) scattering as well as incoherent (Compton) scattering

- One of the major modern databases of photon interaction coefficients should be used, such as NIST (XCOM), EPDL, or PENELOPE

Accurate electron transport in the x-ray target is also critical for accurate x-ray spectral predictions. This transport process determines the number of electrons that are backscattered out of a thick target (or penetrate through a transmission target), as well as the proportion that reaches a given depth and their distributions in energy and direction. These features impact the total x-ray fluence emitted as well as the shape of the energy spectrum [113]. The code system should therefore be well-validated for electron transport in the kilovoltage energy range. Care should also be made to choose appropriate model/transport selections for the energy range, by reference to relevant documentation or publications.

7.3 MONTE CARLO SYSTEMS

Various general-purpose Monte Carlo systems have been developed over the decades. More specialized software is also available for specific applications (e.g. [160, 161]). Software may be free or cost, be open-source or closed-source and the licensing conditions vary. We will focus on widely-available general-purpose code systems here, that are free to use for research purposes. Listed in table 7.1 are some popular systems, sorted alphabetically, that can be used for simulating x-ray tube spectra. Each one of these systems has unique features and solutions for coupled electron-photon transport. The algorithms and physics models implemented are summarized briefly in table 7.2, and further expanded in the following sections dedicated to each system. It is emphasized that the interaction physics and transport mechanisms are described superficially, with more detailed descriptions available in the associated reference manuals, assorted texts on the topic [65, 147, 162], and authoritative reports such as ICRU Report 90 [44].

7.3.1 EGSnrc

EGSnrc is an extension of the EGS (Electron-Gamma-Shower) family of code systems originally developed in the 1970s at the Stanford Linear Accelerator Center (SLAC) for coupled electron-photon transport. However, unlike its predecessor EGS4 [169], the EGSnrc system is maintained by the National Research Council of Canada (NRC). Although it shares certain commonalities with other EGS codes, such as the material data preparation package PEGS4 [169], there are several notable differences. Importantly, EGSnrc is distributed with various applications (sometimes referred to as user codes) developed for source modelling, radiation detector modelling, and radiation dose calculations in medical physics. One such application that is particularly suitable for simulating x-ray tube spectra is BEAMnrc [170]. This application includes a user-friendly front-end interface that has built-in component modules for constructing in detail the main elements of an x-ray tube.

EGSnrc implements a refined electron transport that combines a mixed Class II transport, sometimes called PRESTA-II [171, 172], with single elastic scattering (analogue mode) at geometrical boundaries. The distance from boundaries at which single-event transport is initiated can be specified by the user. An important detail in this is that the BEAMnrc user code artificially displaces boundaries between different regions by a tiny distance to avoid rounding errors. This approach has been shown to introduce considerable

Table 7.1: Popular general-purpose Monte Carlo systems for radiation transport. The programming language is listed along with the (kinetic) energy range for coupled electron-photon transport.

System (release[1])	Language	Energy (eV)	Primary reference
EGSnrc (2021)	Mortran3	10^3–10^{11}	Kawrakow *et al* [163]
FLUKA (2021)	FORTRAN 77	10^3–10^{15}	Ferrari *et al* [164]
Geant4 (2021)	C++	10^2–10^{16}	Agostinelli *et al* [165]
MCNP6 (2018)	Fortran 90	10^2–10^{11}	Goorley *et al* [166]
PENELOPE (2018)	FORTRAN 77	10^2–10^9	Salvat [35]

[1]Release of the latest (current) version at the time of writing

Table 7.2: Summary of the physics implemented in the general-purpose Monte Carlo systems listed in table 7.1. Note that different versions of the Livermore Evaluated Photon-, Electron-, and Atomic Data Libraries (EPDL, EEDL, and EADL) are available, with the most recent update included in the Electron-Photon Interaction Cross Sections (EPICS) library [63].

System	Photon cross sections	Bremsstrahlung energy	Bremsstrahlung angle
EGSnrc	Various options, including EPDL, NIST (XCOM) [167]	Various options, including NIST, NRC (see Section 3.2.1)	KM (eq. 3.10 in eq. 3.9), or SIM (eq. 3.11)
FLUKA	EPDL	NIST	KM
Geant4	Various options, including EPDL, PENELOPE	Various options, including EEDL, NIST	Options include: KQP (eq. 3.7) 2BN (eq. 3.8), 2BS (eq. 3.9)
MCNP6	EPDL	NIST	2BN for $E \lesssim 2$ MeV
PENELOPE	PENELOPE's own database	NIST	KQP

System	Condensed electron transport[1]	Electron impact ionization	Atomic relaxation cascade
EGSnrc	Mixed (Class II) according to energy loss	Various options, including PENELOPE	Detailed or shell-averaged based on EADL atomic data
FLUKA	Mixed (Class II) according to energy loss	Not implemented	Simulated only for ionizations by photon interactions
Geant4	Options include mixed (Class II) according to angle and energy loss	Various options, including EEDL, PENELOPE	Detailed based on atomic data from EADL
MCNP6	Condensed (Class I)	EEDL	Detailed for single-event electron transport (EADL atomic data)
PENELOPE	Mixed (Class II) according to angle and energy loss	Distorted-wave Born approx. by Bote and Salvat [168]	Detailed based on atomic data from EADL

[1]Note that each system has also the option of single-event (analogue) electron transport (described in the text)

errors in the transport of kilovoltage electrons at the surface of solid targets (such as an x-ray tube anode), due to the default size of this boundary adjustment being the same order of magnitude as the electron step size [32]. This issue can, however, be readily resolved by reducing the boundary adjustment distance, as suggested by Ali and Rogers [32].

The photon transport is simulated using an analogue scheme based on sampling from the associated differential cross sections. EGSnrc by default employs the rather obsolete cross sections tabulated by Storm and Israel [173], which are included in the PEGS4 material data. However, more up-to-date evaluations of the photon cross section included in the Livermore EPDL library [63], or the NIST XCOM database [167], can be selected instead. The photoelectric cross section can also be replaced with the renormalized results obtained by Sabatucci and Salvat [174] for the PENELOPE Monte Carlo system (described in Section 7.3.5). Note that a description and comparison of these cross sections can be found in ICRU Report 90 [44].

For the simulation of characteristic x rays it should be noted that previous versions of EGSnrc treated atomic transitions to and from M- and N-shells in an average way, introducing appreciable errors in emission lines for low-energy x-ray sources [175]. However, this functionality has been made obsolete with the introduction of a more detailed atomic relaxation process based on atomic data from the Livermore EADL [63].

A notable feature of the EGSnrc/BEAMnrc system is the advanced variance reduction techniques developed for x-ray source simulations. The Directional Bremsstrahlung Splitting (DBS) technique splits (at the time of creation) the bremsstrahlung photons aimed into a specified field of interest. The complementary Bremsstrahlung Cross Section Enhancement (BCSE) technique scales up the bremsstrahlung production in a material, with a commensurate reduction in the weighting of the photons and implementing randomly decrementing electron energy loss to ensure unbiased results. Optimally combining the BCSE and DBS variance reductions can produce up to five orders of magnitude more efficient x-ray spectra simulations [176].

7.3.2 FLUKA

FLUKA (FLUktuierende KAskade) is a Monte Carlo computer code system developed in the 1960s at the European Organization for Nuclear Research (CERN) for calculating the shielding of high-energy proton accelerators. The current version is the third generation system developed since 1989 with the support of Istituto Nazionale di Fisica Nucleare (INFN). FLUKA has over the years evolved into a powerful multipurpose tool that can simulate the transport of about 60 different particle types over broad ranges of energy. A useful recent addition is the front-end interface FLAIR [177], which facilitates editing of input files, executing simulations, and visualizing the output.

The radiation transport can be simulated in closed-solid bodies and semi-infinite spaces, as well as constructed lattices and voxel geometries.

The transport can be performed in different materials and user-defined electric fields. Due to the many particle types supported, several physics lists (DEFAULTS) have been defined. The physics list for electromagnetic cascades, for example, includes settings (cards) for detailed electron and photon transport. Many additional options can be selected by adding further cards. For instance, single electron scattering (analogue mode) based on Rutherford's formula can be enabled instead of condensed-history tracking based on Molière's multiple-Coulomb-scattering theory [178], as is recommended for low electron energies and high-Z materials (i.e., a typical x-ray target). In order to improve the electron transport at interfaces separating different materials, where the conditions for multiple scattering may not be satisfied, FLUKA has an option for enabling analogue electron transport at geometrical boundaries.

A major disadvantage with the current version of FLUKA is that it lacks subroutines for simulating atomic relaxation following inner-shell ionization by electron impact. Recall from Section 3.3 that electron impact is an important contributor to the fluorescence production in an x-ray tube anode. As such, the characteristic x-ray peaks in simulated x-ray spectra can be substantially underestimated. FLUKA may therefore not be suitable for certain applications that rely on accurate results for the characteristic x-ray emission.

7.3.3 Geant4

The GEANT (GEometry ANd Tracking) series of Monte Carlo systems was, like FLUKA, originally developed at CERN for high-energy physics experiments. The current version, Geant4, has been developed since 1998 by the Geant4 collaboration, which is represented by scientists active at various notable physics laboratories and institutions around the world. It distinguishes itself from most other Monte Carlo systems in that it is based on object-oriented programming. This enables the user to employ powerful methods to manage the computations and makes it possible to add new physics models with little modification to the source code. The code structure includes numerous classes that facilitate all aspects of computation, including the construction of the geometry, execution of the code, and visualization of the tallied results. The geometry can be constructed out of simpler objects built by combining solids defined as three-dimensional primitives, while more intricate geometries can be built in terms of tessellated solids defined by a number of facets. The latter makes it possible to use a geometry constructed in a computer-aided design (CAD) system.

Geant4 provides a large selection of physics models and data for over 100 different particle types. An application can be configured using pre-built physics constructors that initialize a specific physics list. For x-ray simulations there are several electromagnetic (EM) physics constructors available that have been benchmarked for medical physics applications [179]:

G4EmLivermorePhysics
   Implements the Livermore Evaluated Photon-, Electron-, and Atomic

Data libraries (EPDL, EEDL, EADL), for photon interactions, electron ionization (below 100 keV), and atomic relaxation, respectively. These libraries provide a more accurate description of electromagnetic physics in the low-energy range than Geant4's standard sublibraries.

`G4EmPenelopePhysics`

Implements the models and cross sections developed for the PENELOPE Monte Carlo system (described in Section 7.3.5).

`G4EmStandardPhysics_option4`

Implements a combination of physics data and models (including Livermore and PENELOPE) that have been selected based on their perceived performance in terms of accuracy over computational efficiency.

Although these constructors implement the same intrinsic bremsstrahlung energy distribution based on the NIST cross sections by Seltzer and Berger [40, 43], the intrinsic angular distribution differs between them. The PENELOPE physics constructor implements the detailed KQP bremsstrahlung shape function (see Section 3.2.2). The other physics constructors by default sample the bremsstrahlung emission angle from the analytical 2BS formula derived with extreme-relativistic and small-angle approximations. However, the alternative 2BN formula that is better suited for lower-energy applications such as x-ray tube simulations [51], can be selected instead.

The listed physics constructors implement the same mixed Class II condensed-history electron transport described by Kadri *et al* [180], based on Goudsmit-Saunderson angular distribution [181] with the final direction and position of the electron correlated according to Lewis theory [182]. The algorithm combines condensed transport with single-event (analogue) simulations for large-angle deflections. The transport at geometrical boundaries is also analogue. The total elastic-scattering cross section and the transport cross section for single scattering have been generated by the ELSEPA code [183], originally developed for the PENELOPE Monte Carlo system. Inelastic collisions are simulated as discrete events for energy losses exceeding a selected production threshold for secondary particles, otherwise the energy loss is accounted for by the restricted collision stopping power.

Although the object-oriented programming with a plethora of classes and methods makes for an exceptionally powerful code basis, creating your own application can be a daunting task. It is, however worth noting that for those who prefer to work with a simpler macro-based programming language, the platform GATE [184] might be a useful alternative. GATE is an open-source Monte Carlo simulation platform that encapsulates the Geant4 libraries. It has been developed by the international OpenGATE collaboration specifically for medical physics applications and includes an impressive set of tools for various x-ray imaging, nuclear medicine, and radiotherapy simulations.

7.3.4 MCNP6

MCNP (Monte Carlo N-Particle) is a family of Monte Carlo code systems developed at the Los Alamos National Laboratory (LANL). The history of developing Monte Carlo techniques at LANL dates back to the late 1940s, when statistical methods were applied to solve neutron diffusion problems in fission devices using the first generation of electronic computers. Major methodological and technological progress since then have made possible the development of MCNP6, a Monte Carlo code system that can transport about 40 different particle types over broad ranges of energies. The simulation geometry can be constructed from arbitrary three-dimensional cells containing user-defined materials bounded by first- and second-degree surfaces and fourth-degree elliptical tori. MCNP6 can also simulate the transport in meshed geometries generated by a Computer Aided Engineering (CAE) software.

It is worth noting that MCNP6 differs considerably from its predecessors in both the algorithms and the data libraries used for coupled electron-photon transport [185], making it better suited for simulating kilovoltage x-ray spectra. For instance, MCNP6 includes new sources of atomic data (EPICS2014 [63]) that allow for the full detailed relaxation cascade to be computed rather than the average K- and L-shell transitions, as was the case with the previous MCNPX [186] and MCNP5 codes [187].

MCNP6 implements a Class I condensed-history algorithm similar to that of the Integrated TIGER Series (ITS) [188], as described by Hughes [189]. This algorithm simulates the movement of the electrons in steps long enough to encompass many collisions, but short enough that the underlying Gaudsmit-Saunderson theory for angular deflections [181] and Landau theory [190] for energy-loss straggling (with enhancements by Blunck-Leisegang [191]) remain valid. The step length has been defined as the distance for an electron to lose a fraction of its energy in the continuous-slowing-down approximation (CSDA), with a number of substeps determined empirically for each element to optimize accuracy and efficiency [192]. In addition to the condensed approach, a single-event (analogue) algorithm that relies on the associated differential cross sections is activated for electron transport below user-specified energy (1 keV by default). This is an important feature for x-ray spectra simulations given that the implemented condensed-history algorithm neglects fluorescence caused by electron impact ionization of L, M, and higher shells [193]. Hence, more accurate calculations of the characteristic x-ray emission can be achieved by enabling the single-event electron transport for the entire range of simulated energies [129].

7.3.5 PENELOPE

PENELOPE (PENetration and Energy LOss of Positrons and Electrons) is a code system for Monte Carlo simulation of coupled electron-photon transport developed at the Universitat de Barcelona since 1996 for distribution by the OECD Nuclear Energy Agency Data Bank. It is known particularly for its state-of-the-art numerical databases and analytical models for low-energy interaction mechanisms. PENELOPE uses a set of subroutines that are called PENGEOM [194] to track particles through material structures composed of homogeneous geometrical bodies limited by quadric surfaces, such as planes, spheres, cylinders, and cones. A separate subroutine is available for the simulation of charged particle transport under external static electric (and magnetic) fields.

A simulation is configured by a user code, such as penEasy [195,196], which provides a number of additional features, including seamless transport in mixed quadric-voxelized geometries, several types of tallies to score quantities of interest, and extended capabilities of variance reduction techniques. One such variance reduction technique is interaction forcing, which can be used to artificially increase the bremsstrahlung production in the x-ray target.

PENELOPE implements a mixed Class II electron transport that simulates *soft* interactions by means of condensed-history tracking, while *hard* elastic collisions, inelastic collisions, and bremsstrahlung interactions are simulated in detail. Hard events are those involving angular deflections or energy losses that exceed certain cutoffs and are simulated individually based on the associated differential cross sections. Soft collisions are simulated according to the random-hinge method [197]: the effects of all soft collisions between consecutive hard interactions are combined into a single artificial event (a hinge), simulated at a random position along the track. This method is able to simulate multiple-scattering processes in both extended homogeneous bodies and in complex geometries with multiple material interfaces [35]. Note that the parameters specifying the cutoffs for hard or soft events can be set to treat all interactions as hard events, in which case the entire electron transport is performed in analogue mode.

Similar to the other Monte Carlo systems covered in this chapter, the photon transport is realized using a detailed (analogue) scheme that simulates the interactions in chronological succession based on the associated differential cross sections. What separates PENELOPE from the other systems is that it uses its own database of cross sections. A recent survey of photon cross sections performed by Cullen [198] indicates that PENELOPE differs from NIST (XCOM) and recent versions of EPDL (EPICS2014 and EPICS2017) generally by a few percent in the kilovoltage energy range due to the photoelectric cross section. These results are consistent with differences observed in Monte Carlo-calculated macroscopic quantities such as the mass energy-absorption coefficient [199,200], which is a quantity relevant for radiation dosimetry and beam-quality characterization as outlined in Chapter 4.

PENELOPE uses photoelectric subshell cross sections generated with the program PHOTACS [174], which uses the same theory as the calculations of Scofield [201] implemented in XCOM and EPDL, but with a screening normalization correction factor applied to account for inaccuracies in the atomic wave function used [202,203]. It should be noted that in their original calculations, Scofield also provided such factors for a limited range of elements, and that earlier compilations of cross sections used the renormalized Scofield results [204]. Nevertheless, this kind of correction is somewhat controversial given that comparisons with experimental measurements are scarce and appear to be contradictory, as reported by ICRU 90 [44], which gives no formal recommendation on this matter. It is emphasized that more recent versions of PENELOPE include an alternative database of photoelectric cross sections generated without the screening normalization correction.

Another set of cross sections originally developed for the PENELOPE Monte Carlo systems are those for inner-shell electron impact ionization. Recall from Section 3.3 that electron impact directly influences the production of characteristic x rays. In fact, using different methods for the electron impact and the subsequent relaxation cascade has been shown to produce considerable differences in the resulting characteristic x-ray lines [113, 193]. The PENELOPE cross sections are based on quantum mechanical calculations in the distorted-wave (first) Born approximation and the plane-wave (first) Born approximation (PWBA theory) for low and high initial electron energies, respectively [168]; this model has been extensively validated against experimental results, indicating good agreement [61]. It is emphasized that these cross sections have also been made available in several of the other Monte Carlo systems covered in this chapter (see table 7.2).

There is no Python related content for this chapter. A good way to start with modelling x-ray tubes using the Monte Carlo method is to download the EGSnrc code system and use the BEAMnrc user code (https://nrc-cnrc.github.io/EGSnrc/). The input file for the example tube illustrated in fig. 2.5 is included in this book's software repository, at https://bitbucket.org/caxtus, along with the associated PEGS4 material data file.

III

Applications

CHAPTER 8

Predicting and matching half-value layers

T HIS chapter discusses the issues to consider when predicting or matching beam-quality metrics such as half-value layer and illustrates the points with a comparison between measurements by three Primary Standards Dosimetry Laboratories and predictions of a spectrum model.

8.1 INTRODUCTION

Perhaps the most commonly measured and modelled metric of beam quality is the half-value layer (HVL). The first and second HVL, together, give a good indication of the penetrative characteristics of an x-ray beam. It is straightforward to obtain estimates using the spectrum calculation software discussed in this book (see Chapter 5). When predictions do not agree with expectations, however, it is often troublesome to identify the source of the problem: is it the measurements, the spectrum model, or the input selections for the model that are at fault?

In some circumstances, when there is a minor disagreement between model predictions and the desired beam quality (a few percent), the input parameters to the model can simply be adjusted in an *ad hoc* manner to produce the required result. This can be done, for example, by "tweaking" the thickness of the filtration. In other situations this is unsatisfactory and the root cause of the discrepancy needs to be identified. Below we highlight some issues to consider.

8.1.1 Filtration

Ideally, full information on filtration would be available from the manufacturer. However, both inherent and added filtration are often stated as an aluminium-equivalent thickness. This is a nominal value valid at a specific tube potential (which should be stated). In reality, the inherent filtration may consist of a combination of oil, glass, beryllium, and, possibly, actually

DOI: 10.1201/9781003058168-8

aluminium. The added filtration often involves aluminium and copper but may include tin and many other materials.

Even if the actual materials are all specified, this may be at low accuracy. A stated 0.1 mm of copper filtration, for example, may leave a substantial uncertainty on its precise thickness.

The use of metal alloys in filters may also lead to uncertainties in composition. And even if the stated material is an element, it must be considered whether it can be assumed to be a *pure* element. When we come across "aluminium" in every-day life, for example, it is rarely pure aluminium, due to its inferior mechanical properties.

8.1.2 Anode angle and tube tilt

Information on the tube geometry may be available in documentation from the manufacturer. The anode angle should be established if possible and any tube tilt. If the whole tube *is* tilted with respect to the central axis of the beam (see fig. 2.4), the filtration itself may also be tilted. If so, the oblique path-length of x-rays through the filtration will be longer than the filter thickness.

When using modelling software, it should be clarified what value of anode angle is assumed and whether it is adjustable. The interpretation of the predictions should also be clarified e.g. whether the result is valid for the central axis, or averaged over an area.

8.1.3 Tube potential

Often we are obliged to simply assume that the nominal selected tube potential is accurate. However, if the tube is assessed in regular Quality Control (QC) tests, there may be information available on the likely accuracy of the nominal selections.

In modern tubes, with high-frequency generators, the assumption that the x-ray exposure is conducted at constant potential is often reasonable. If information is available on the voltage ripple, however, and it proves to be substantial, it may need to be modelled (see Section 2.2.1).

8.1.4 Measurement conditions

The detector or dosimeter, such as an ionization chamber, should be appropriate for the energy range of the measurements. Other issues to consider are:

• Were the measurements made close to the central axis, or displaced in the anode-cathode or the orthogonal direction?

• Is the source-to-detector distance well-known?

• What size is the sensitive volume or area of the detector?

- Can the measurements be considered to be under the narrow-beam conditions appropriate to most x-ray models? That is, can the scattered x-ray fluence reaching the detector be considered negligible?

- Could any of the filtration generate characteristic radiation that would reach the detector and affect the results?

- What are the compositions of any attenuators used for half-value layer determination e.g. are they high-purity aluminium or an alloy such as Aluminium 1100?

- At what angle do the x rays strike the detector? If they strike a flat detector at an oblique angle, the number of x rays entering the sensitive area is reduced with the cosine of the angle (see eq. (4.2) and the discussion of planar fluence)

8.1.5 Air column

Almost invariably, there is a column of air present between the tube exit window and the detector. The density of air is low (about 0.001 g cm^{-3}) and often it has a negligible effect on the beam quality and causes only a small reduction on the detected fluence. The cumulative effect of many centimetres of air can be significant, however, particularly for spectra generated with low tube potentials and light filtration. When uncertain of its importance, the air column should be included in any spectrum model.

8.1.6 Tube ageing

Tube performance often changes over a tube's lifetime. Over time, vapour liberated from the target can accumulate on the tube exit window. The anode surface can also become pitted or roughen. Both these phenomena increase the effective inherent filtration.

8.2 BENCHMARK SPECTRUM SPECIFICATIONS

Experimental results published by Primary Standards Dosimetry Laboratories must be considered some of the most reliable measurements available. This makes them ideal for comparison with predictions from models. Obtaining sufficient information regarding the measurements conditions, however, is not always easy, as some details may not be included in published reports or listed on laboratory websites.

The information presented in tables 8.1 and 8.2 for standard spectra of the Physikalisch-Technische Bundesanstalt (PTB; Braunschweig, Germany) was derived from a report by the institute [20]. The RQR and RQA beams provided in table 8.1 represent typical diagnostic x-ray beam qualities emitted from a minimally-filtered tube, and, after attenuation by a patient,

Table 8.1: Specifications for the IEC RQR/RQA beam spectra [145] of Physikalisch-Technische Bundesanstalt (PTB) [20]. The first and second half-value layers (HVL$_1$ and HVL$_2$) are specified at 100 cm. A monitor chamber was also present in the beam (0.25 mm Kapton).

Name	Tube pot'l [kV]	Filtration Be [mm]	Filtration Al [mm]	HVL$_1$ [mm Al]	HVL$_2$ [mm Al]
RQR2	40	1	2.5	1.36	1.72
RQR3	50	1	2.5	1.72	2.30
RQR4	60	1	2.5	2.02	2.84
RQR5	70	1	2.5	2.29	3.37
RQR6	80	1	2.5	2.59	3.96
RQR7	90	1	2.5	2.91	4.57
RQR8	100	1	2.5	3.23	5.19
RQR9	120	1	2.5	3.88	6.37
RQR10	150	7	2.5	5.01	8.15
RQA2	40	1	6.5	2.13	2.41
RQA3	50	1	12.5	3.67	4.05
RQA4	60	1	18.5	5.24	5.70
RQA5	70	1	23.5	6.64	7.16
RQA6	80	1	28.5	7.96	8.50
RQA7	90	1	32.5	9.03	9.57
RQA8	100	1	36.5	9.93	10.47
RQA9	120	1	42.5	11.37	11.97
RQA10	150	7	50.0	12.97	13.66

respectively [69]. The beam qualities provided in table 8.2 represent high kerma-rate (H), wide-spectra (W), narrow-spectra (N), and low kerma-rate (L) beams [145]. Broadly, these can be interpreted as beams with low-filtration, low homogeneity coefficient, high homogeneity coefficient, and high filtration, respectively. Measurements with a tube potential of 120 kV or below were performed with an AEG MB 121/1 x-ray tube with inherent filtration of 1 mm Be. Other measurements were performed with an AEG 420/1 tube with inherent filtration of 7 mm Be. The uncertainties on the tube potentials of the two tubes were 10 V and 100 V, respectively. Both tubes had an anode angle of 20°. A monitor chamber was present (0.25 mm Kapton Polyimide film). The purity of the filter materials was 99.98% (Al) or 99.99% (Cu, Sn, Pb). The source-to-detector distance was 100 cm in a narrow-beam geometry. The spectra were measured with a high-purity germanium (HPGe) detector. Half-value layers were calculated from the measured spectra using unrenormalized photon cross sections.

Equivalent spectra to table 8.2 are also produced by the National Institute of Standards and Technology (NIST; Gaithersburg, MD, USA) and denoted HK/WS/NS/LK [205]. The information is presented in table 8.3 and specified for a Comet MR320/26 tube with Pantak generator (3 mm Be window, 20°

Table 8.2: Specifications for the ISO H/W/N/L beam spectra [69] of Physikalisch-Technische Bundesanstalt (PTB) [20]. The first and second half-value layers (HVL_1 and HVL_2) are specified at 100 cm. A monitor chamber was also present in the beam (0.25 mm Kapton).

Name	Tube pot'l [kV]	Be [mm]	Al [mm]	Filtration Cu [mm]	Sn [mm]	Pb [mm]	HVL_1 [mm Cu]	HVL_2 [mm Cu]
H60	60	1.0	3.9	0.0	0.0	0.0	0.0839	0.121
H100	100	1.0	4.0	0.15	0.0	0.0	0.294	0.462
H200	200	7.0	4.0	1.0	0.0	0.0	1.54	2.28
H250	250	7.0	4.0	1.60	0.0	0.0	2.42	3.24
H280	280	7.0	4.0	3.0	0.0	0.0	3.26	3.88
H300	300	7.0	4.0	2.2	0.0	0.0	3.22	4.00
W60	60	1.0	4.0	0.3	0.0	0.0	0.18	0.215
W80	80	1.0	4.0	0.5	0.0	0.0	0.349	0.433
W110	110	1.0	4.0	2.0	0.0	0.0	0.933	1.08
W150	150	7.0	4.0	0.0	1.0	0.0	1.78	2.03
W200	150	7.0	4.0	0.0	2.0	0.0	3.00	3.24
W250	250	7.0	4.0	0.0	4.0	0.0	4.14	4.34
W300	300	7.0	4.0	0.0	6.5	0.0	5.03	5.18
N40	40	1.0	4.0	0.21	0.0	0.0	0.085	0.0927
N60	60	1.0	4.0	0.6	0.0	0.0	0.234	0.263
N80	80	1.0	4.0	2.0	0.0	0.0	0.578	0.622
N100	100	1.0	4.0	5.0	0.0	0.0	1.09	1.15
N120	120	1.0	4.0	5.0	1.0	0.0	1.67	1.73
N150	150	7.0	4.0	0.0	2.5	0.0	2.30	2.41
N200	200	7.0	4.0	2.0	3.0	1.0	3.92	3.99
N250	250	7.0	4.0	0.0	2.0	3.0	5.10	5.14
N300	300	7.0	4.0	0.0	3.0	5.0	5.96	6.00
L55	55	1.0	4.0	1.2	0.0	0.0	0.248	0.261
L70	70	1.0	4.0	2.5	0.0	0.0	0.483	0.505
L100	100	1.0	4.0	0.5	2.0	0.0	1.22	1.25
L125	125	7.0	4.0	1.0	4.0	0.0	1.98	2.02
L170	170	7.0	4.0	1.0	3.0	1.5	3.40	3.46
L210	210	7.0	4.0	0.5	2.0	3.5	4.52	4.55
L240	240	7.0	4.0	0.5	2.0	5.5	5.19	5.22

anode angle, potential adjustable to 100 V). Half-value layers were determined by the attenuation of air kerma. NIST use only high-purity materials for the filters and half-value layer measurements, with the purity of the copper used for the latter being 99.9%[1]. The source-to-detector distance was 100 cm with a narrow-beam geometry appropriate for half-value layer determinations.

Information for the reference spectra of the International Bureau of Weights and Measures (BIPM) for tube potentials from 23 to 250 kV are

---

[1]Private communication with C.M. O'Brien at NIST during the work presented in ref. [1].

Table 8.3: Specifications for the ISO H/W/N/L beam spectra [208] of National Institute of Standards and Technology (NIST) [205]. The first and second half-value layers (HVL_1 and HVL_2) are specified at 100 cm. The filtration due to the x-ray tube's Be window is included in the stated (equivalent) Al filtration.

Name	Tube pot'l [kV]	Be [mm]	Al [mm]	Cu [mm]	Sn [mm]	Pb [mm]	HVL_1 [mm Cu]	HVL_2 [mm Cu]
HK60	60	0.0	3.19	0.0	0.0	0.0	0.079	0.113
HK100	100	0.0	3.9	0.15	0.0	0.0	0.298	0.463
HK200	200	0.0	4.0	1.15	0.0	0.0	1.669	2.447
HK250	250	0.0	4.0	1.60	0.0	0.0	2.463	3.37
HK280	280	0.0	4.0	3.06	0.0	0.0	3.493	4.089
HK300	300	0.0	4.0	2.51	0.0	0.0	3.474	4.205
WS60	60	0.0	4.0	0.3	0.0	0.0	0.179	0.206
WS80	80	0.0	4.0	0.529	0.0	0.0	0.337	0.44
WS110	110	0.0	4.0	2.029	0.0	0.0	0.97	1.13
WS150	150	0.0	4.0	0.0	1.03	0.0	1.88	2.13
WS200	150	0.0	4.0	0.0	2.01	0.0	3.09	3.35
WS250	250	0.0	4.0	0.0	4.01	0.0	4.30	4.5
WS300	300	0.0	4.0	0.0	6.54	0.0	5.23	5.38
NS40	40	0.0	4.0	0.21	0.0	0.0	0.082	0.094
NS60	60	0.0	4.0	0.6	0.0	0.0	0.241	0.271
NS80	80	0.0	4.0	2.0	0.0	0.0	0.59	0.62
NS100	100	0.0	4.0	5.0	0.0	0.0	1.14	1.19
NS120	120	0.0	4.0	4.99	1.04	0.0	1.76	1.84
NS150	150	0.0	4.0	0.0	2.5	0.0	2.41	2.57
NS200	200	0.0	4.0	2.04	2.98	1.003	4.09	4.20
NS250	250	0.0	4.0	0.0	2.01	2.97	5.34	5.40
NS300	300	0.0	4.0	0.0	2.99	4.99	6.17	6.30
LK55	55	0.0	4.0	1.19	0.0	0.0	0.260	-
LK70	70	0.0	4.0	2.64	0.0	0.0	0.509	-
LK100	100	0.0	4.0	0.52	2.0	0.0	1.27	-
LK125	125	0.0	4.0	1.0	4.0	0.0	2.107	2.094
LK170	170	0.0	4.0	1.0	3.0	1.5	3.565	3.592
LK210	210	0.0	4.0	0.5	2.0	3.5	4.726	4.733
LK240	240	0.0	4.0	0.5	2.0	5.5	5.515	5.542

collected in table 8.4. Two tungsten target x-ray tubes are used at BIPM for such determinations–Comet MXR-160/21 and MXR-320/26 tubes–both with a $20°$ anode angle[2]. These are operated at constant potential with a high stability generator. Inherent filtration was considered to be 3 mm Be [206]. Half-value layers were determined by attenuation of air kerma and high purity filters (>99.9%) were used [207]. The reference plane for measurements was

---

[2]Private communication with C. Kessler at BIPM during the writing of this book.

50 cm from the tube exit window (≤ 50 kV) or 120 cm from the source (>50 kV).

For the PTB and NIST spectra referenced, it was assumed that a column of air (dry, at sea level) of 95 cm was present. For the BIPM spectra, 50 cm or 115 cm of air (dry, at sea level) was assumed. All spectra modelled in this chapter were calculated with SpekPy-v2 (kqp) [2]. The physics model selection of "kqp" indicates that the full spectrum model described in Chapter 6 was used.

Table 8.4: Specifications for the reference beams of the International Bureau of Weights and Measures (BIPM) [206]. The first half-value layers (HVL$_1$) are specified in mm of Al and/or Cu. The reference planes were at 50 cm (from the exit window) for tube potentials below 100 kV and at a source-to-detector distance of 120 cm otherwise.

Name	Tube pot'l [kV]	Be [mm]	Filtration Al [mm]	Cu [mm]	Mo [mm]	HVL$_1$ [mm Al]	HVL$_1$ [mm Cu]
BIPM30	30	3.0	0.208	0.0	0.0	0.169	–
BIPM25	25	3.0	0.372	0.0	0.0	0.242	–
BIPM50a	50	3.0	1.008	0.0	0.0	1.017	–
BIPM50b	50	3.0	3.989	0.0	0.0	2.262	–
BIPM23M	23	3.0	0.0	0.0	0.06	0.332	–
BIPM25M	25	3.0	0.0	0.0	0.06	0.342	–
BIPM28M	28	3.0	0.0	0.0	0.06	0.355	–
BIPM30M	30	3.0	0.0	0.0	0.06	0.364	–
BIPM35M	35	3.0	0.0	0.0	0.06	0.388	–
BIPM40M	50	3.0	0.0	0.0	0.06	0.417	–
BIPM50M	50	3.0	0.0	0.0	0.06	0.489	–
BIPM100	100	3.0	3.431	0.0	0.0	4.030	0.149
BIPM135	135	3.0	2.228	0.232	0.0	–	0.489
BIPM180	180	3.0	2.228	0.485	0.0	–	0.977
BIPM250	250	3.0	2.228	1.570	0.0	–	2.484

8.3 PREDICTING AND MATCHING HALF-VALUE LAYERS

To illustrate the standard beam qualities, five spectra specified at 100 kV tube potential are shown in fig. 8.1. The HVL$_1$ values vary between 0.12 and 1.22 mm Cu. Tube potential alone obviously does not adequately specify beam quality. Figure 8.2 shows six very different standard spectra modified with copper filtration to produce an HVL$_1$ of precisely 0.3 mm Cu. The tube potentials and homogeneity coefficients ($h_i = $ HVL$_1$/HVL$_2$) vary widely. The first half-value layer, therefore, is also inadequate by itself in uniquely specifying beam quality. Indicating the tube potential *and* HVL$_1$ is an improvement, but specifying both HVL$_1$ and HVL$_2$ is probably better still (see Chapter 4, in particular Section 4.2.2).

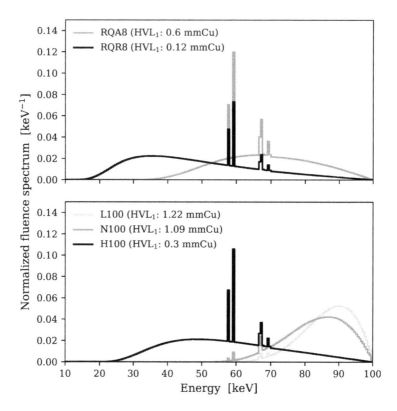

Figure 8.1: Five standard spectra (RQR8, RQA8, H100, N100, L100) specified for a 100 kV tube potential. The spectra were calculated with SpekPy-v2 (kqp) with PTB filtration specifications [20].

A comparison with the reference first and second half-value layers in mm of aluminium is presented in table 8.5 for the IEC spectra (RQR/RQA). The mean $\pm$ standard deviation in the discrepancies for HVL_1 and HVL_2 were $1.2\pm0.5\%$ and $0.2\pm0.4\%$, respectively[3]. The additional thickness of aluminium that would be required to exactly match the reference first half-value layer is also tabulated. For most beam qualities, this is a small adjustment.

The results for the H/W/N/L spectra of PTB and NIST are presented in tables 8.6 and 8.7. For the PTB spectra, the mean $\pm$ standard deviation in the discrepancies for HVL_1 and HVL_2 were $0.8\pm0.8\%$ and $0.4\pm0.6\%$, respectively. For the NIST spectra, the mean and standard deviations in the discrepancies

---

[3]Note that the default selection in SpekPy (kqp) is to use renormalized photon cross sections. In the PTB reference, unrenormalized cross sections were used for calculating half-value layers. Selecting the same in SpekPy, for consistency, the discrepancies become: $0.6 \pm 0.5\%$ and $-0.3 \pm 0.4\%$ for the first and second half-value layers, respectively.

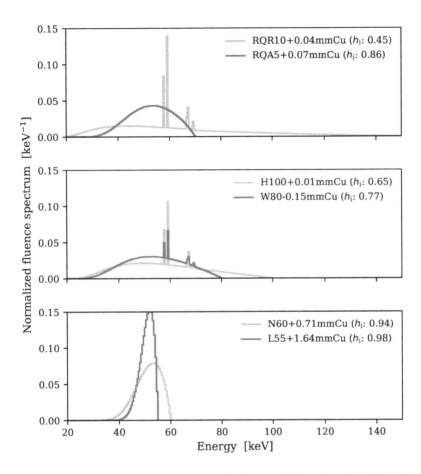

Figure 8.2: Six modified standard spectra (RQR10, RQA5, H100, W80, N60, L55) with a first half-value layer of 0.3 mm Cu. The amount of Cu filtration added or subtracted to match the half-value layer is displayed, along with the resulting homogeneity coefficient (h_i). The spectra were calculated with SpekPy-v2 (kqp) with PTB filtration specifications [20].

for HVL_1 and HVL_2 were $-2.7 \pm 2.4\%$ and $-3.0 \pm 2.0\%$, respectively. We emphasize that not only did the two institutes use different x-ray tubes, they also used different methods of determining half-value layer: the PTB reference values were based on measured spectra, while the NIST values were based on air kerma measurements.

For the BIPM reference spectra (see table 8.8), also based on dosimetry rather than spectrometry, the mean and standard deviations in discrepancies with SpekPy predictions were $-1.6 \pm 0.6\%$ for HVL_1.

Overall, it is not clear whether the predictions of SpekPy differ from the experimental determinations of the Primary Standards Dosimetry

Table 8.5: Predictions for the first and second half-value layers (HVL_1 and HVL_2) for IEC RQR/RQA beam spectra [145] of Physikalisch-Technische Bundesanstalt (PTB) [20] compared to published reference values. Predicted values were calculated with SpekPy-v2 (kqp). The additional required thickness of aluminium to exactly match the reference first HVL is also provided.

Name	Ref. HVL_1 [mm Al]	Pred. HVL_1 [mm Al]		Ref. HVL_2 [mm Al]	Pred. HVL_2 [mm Al]		Req. thick. [mm]
RQR2	1.36	1.387	(2.0%)	1.72	1.724	(0.2%)	-0.09
RQR3	1.72	1.737	(1.0%)	2.30	2.301	(0.0%)	-0.04
RQR4	2.02	2.044	(1.2%)	2.84	2.845	(0.2%)	-0.05
RQR5	2.29	2.327	(1.6%)	3.37	3.370	(0.0%)	-0.07
RQR6	2.59	2.629	(1.5%)	3.96	3.951	(-0.2%)	-0.06
RQR7	2.91	2.948	(1.3%)	4.57	4.567	(-0.1%)	-0.06
RQR8	3.23	3.273	(1.3%)	5.19	5.182	(-0.2%)	-0.06
RQR9	3.88	3.944	(1.7%)	6.37	6.379	(0.1%)	-0.07
RQR10	5.01	5.080	(1.4%)	8.15	8.125	(-0.3%)	-0.07
RQA2	2.13	2.161	(1.5%)	2.41	2.415	(0.2%)	-0.23
RQA3	3.67	3.712	(1.1%)	4.05	4.067	(0.4%)	-0.38
RQA4	5.24	5.261	(0.4%)	5.70	5.701	(0.0%)	-0.22
RQA5	6.64	6.655	(0.2%)	7.16	7.165	(0.1%)	-0.16
RQA6	7.96	8.008	(0.6%)	8.50	8.543	(0.5%)	-0.61
RQA7	9.03	9.082	(0.6%)	9.57	9.610	(0.4%)	-0.75
RQA8	9.93	9.992	(0.6%)	10.47	10.514	(0.4%)	-1.01
RQA9	11.37	11.437	(0.6%)	11.97	11.988	(0.2%)	-1.21
RQA10	12.97	13.261	(2.2%)	13.66	13.859	(1.5%)	-5.36

Laboratories to any greater extent than the laboratories do from each other. It has been suggested that if the first and second half-value layers of two x-ray beams both agree with ±5%, then they can be assumed to be of the same quality [69]. Judged against this standard, the SpekPy model performs well, rarely failing to meet this requirement. While the 5% rule may be a reasonable "rule of thumb", it is important to remember that the accuracy required in modelling spectra is task dependent [208].

With any spectrum model, where a discrepancy with a measured HVL_1 is apparent, a reasonable strategy may be to simply adjust the model's filtration to provide improved agreement. However, it should be borne in mind that, as clearly demonstrated in fig. 8.2, the first half-value layer alone cannot uniquely specify a beam quality.

Table 8.6: Predictions for the first and second half-value layers (HVL$_1$ and HVL$_2$) for ISO H/W/N/L beam spectra [69] of Physikalisch-Technische Bundesanstalt (PTB) [20] compared to published reference values. Predicted values were calculated with SpekPy-v2 (kqp).

Name	Ref. HVL$_1$ [mm Cu]	Pred. HVL$_1$ [mm Cu]		Ref. HVL$_2$ [mm Cu]	Pred. HVL$_2$ [mm Cu]	
H60	0.0839	0.086	(2.0%)	0.121	0.121	(-0.3%)
H100	0.294	0.296	(0.7%)	0.462	0.461	(-0.2%)
H200	1.54	1.566	(1.7%)	2.28	2.296	(0.7%)
H250	2.42	2.467	(2.0%)	3.24	3.266	(0.8%)
H280	3.26	3.340	(2.5%)	3.88	3.925	(1.2%)
H300	3.22	3.261	(1.3%)	4.0	4.009	(0.2%)
W60	0.18	0.182	(0.9%)	0.215	0.216	(0.3%)
W80	0.349	0.350	(0.2%)	0.433	0.432	(-0.2%)
W110	0.933	0.934	(0.1%)	1.08	1.078	(-0.2%)
W150	1.78	1.816	(2.0%)	2.03	2.057	(1.3%)
W200	3.0	3.040	(1.3%)	3.24	3.265	(0.8%)
W250	4.14	4.181	(1.0%)	4.34	4.359	(0.4%)
W300	5.03	5.073	(0.9%)	5.18	5.220	(0.8%)
N40	0.085	0.085	(-0.5%)	0.0927	0.092	(-0.8%)
N60	0.234	0.233	(-0.3%)	0.263	0.261	(-0.9%)
N80	0.578	0.576	(-0.3%)	0.622	0.620	(-0.4%)
N100	1.09	1.095	(0.5%)	1.15	1.153	(0.3%)
N120	1.67	1.684	(0.9%)	1.73	1.748	(1.0%)
N150	2.3	2.324	(1.1%)	2.41	2.435	(1.0%)
N200	3.92	3.943	(0.6%)	3.99	4.008	(0.5%)
N250	5.1	5.138	(0.8%)	5.14	5.181	(0.8%)
N300	5.96	6.040	(1.4%)	6.0	6.071	(1.2%)
L55	0.248	0.247	(-0.5%)	0.261	0.259	(-0.7%)
L70	0.483	0.482	(-0.2%)	0.505	0.503	(-0.3%)
L100	1.22	1.216	(-0.4%)	1.25	1.254	(0.4%)
L125	1.98	2.005	(1.3%)	2.02	2.045	(1.2%)
L170	3.4	3.426	(0.8%)	3.46	3.480	(0.6%)
L210	4.52	4.541	(0.5%)	4.55	4.571	(0.5%)
L240	5.19	5.248	(1.1%)	5.22	5.268	(0.9%)

Table 8.7: Predictions for the first and second half-value layers (HVL$_1$ and HVL$_2$) for ISO H/W/N/L beam spectra [208] of National Institute of Standards and Technology (NIST) [205] compared to published reference values. Predicted values were calculated with SpekPy-v2 (kqp).

Name	Ref. HVL$_1$ [mm Cu]	Pred. HVL$_1$ [mm Cu]		Ref. HVL$_2$ [mm Cu]	Pred. HVL$_2$ [mm Cu]	
HK60	0.079	0.075	(-4.8%)	0.113	0.109	(-3.8%)
HK100	0.298	0.293	(-1.6%)	0.463	0.458	(-1.1%)
HK200	1.669	1.642	(-1.6%)	2.447	2.347	(-4.1%)
HK250	2.463	2.438	(-1.0%)	3.37	3.243	(-3.8%)
HK280	3.493	3.332	(-4.6%)	4.089	3.914	(-4.3%)
HK300	3.474	3.350	(-3.6%)	4.205	4.044	(-3.8%)
WS60	0.179	0.181	(1.3%)	0.206	0.215	(4.6%)
WS80	0.337	0.358	(6.1%)	0.44	0.439	(-0.3%)
WS110	0.97	0.938	(-3.3%)	1.13	1.082	(-4.3%)
WS150	1.88	1.827	(-2.8%)	2.13	2.064	(-3.1%)
WS200	3.09	3.034	(-1.8%)	3.35	3.260	(-2.7%)
WS250	4.3	4.174	(-2.9%)	4.5	4.353	(-3.3%)
WS300	5.23	5.069	(-3.1%)	5.38	5.215	(-3.1%)
NS40	0.082	0.085	(3.1%)	0.094	0.092	(-2.2%)
NS60	0.241	0.233	(-3.3%)	0.271	0.261	(-3.8%)
NS80	0.59	0.576	(-2.4%)	0.62	0.619	(-0.1%)
NS100	1.14	1.095	(-4.0%)	1.19	1.153	(-3.1%)
NS120	1.76	1.690	(-4.0%)	1.84	1.752	(-4.8%)
NS150	2.41	2.321	(-3.7%)	2.57	2.432	(-5.4%)
NS200	4.09	3.940	(-3.7%)	4.2	4.006	(-4.6%)
NS250	5.34	5.131	(-3.9%)	5.4	5.175	(-4.2%)
NS300	6.17	6.037	(-2.2%)	6.3	6.068	(-3.7%)
LK55	0.26	0.246	(-5.3%)	-	0.259	-
LK70	0.509	0.489	(-4.0%)	-	0.509	-
LK100	1.27	1.216	(-4.2%)	-	1.255	-
LK125	2.107	2.004	(-4.9%)	2.094	2.044	(-2.4%)
LK170	3.565	3.424	(-4.0%)	3.592	3.478	(-3.2%)
LK210	4.726	4.540	(-3.9%)	4.733	4.570	(-3.5%)
LK240	5.515	5.247	(-4.9%)	5.542	5.266	(-5.0%)

Table 8.8: Predictions for the first half-value layers (HVL_1) of the International Bureau of Weights and Measures (BIPM) reference spectra compared to published reference values in mm of Al and/or Cu [206]. Predicted values were calculated with SpekPy-v2 (kqp).

Name	Ref. HVL_1 [mm Al]	Pred. HVL_1 [mm Al]		Ref. HVL_1 [mm Cu]	Pred. HVL_1 [mm Cu]
BIPM30	0.169	0.166	(-1.8%)	-	-
BIPM25	0.242	0.238	(-1.8%)	-	-
BIPM50a	1.017	1.005	(-1.2%)	-	-
BIPM50b	2.262	2.225	(-1.6%)	-	-
BIPM23M	0.332	0.326	(-1.7%)	-	-
BIPM25M	0.342	0.338	(-1.3%)	-	-
BIPM28M	0.355	0.350	(-1.3%)	-	-
BIPM30M	0.364	0.359	(-1.4%)	-	-
BIPM35M	0.388	0.383	(-1.3%)	-	-
BIPM40M	0.417	0.412	(-1.3%)	-	-
BIPM50M	0.489	0.484	(-1.1%)	-	-
BIPM100	4.030	3.950	(-2.0%)	0.149	0.147 (-1.1%)
BIPM135	-	-		0.489	0.481 (-1.7%)
BIPM180	-	-		0.977	0.960 (-1.8%)
BIPM250	-	-		2.484	2.397 (-3.5%)

The Python scripts used for generating the data of tables 8.5 to 8.8 are available in the repository to this book, at https://bitbucket.org/caxtus. The scripts are called *beams_ptb_iec.py*, *beams_ptb_iso.py*, *beams_nist_iso.py* and *beams_bipm.py* and use the SpekPy-v2 toolkit. In the scripts, the physics model of SpekPy is set to the most advanced: "kqp". Try changing this to "spekcalc" in *beams_bipm.py* and running the script. Where does the SpekCalc model perform poorly and why? Note that this model does not include L-lines in the characteristic spectrum.

Hint: see Section 5.4 for a discussion of the performance of SpekCalc and other models.

CHAPTER 9

Kilovoltage x-ray beam dosimetry

B ASIC quantities and concepts on the dosimetry of kilovoltage x rays have been presented in Chapter 4. Given an x-ray beam, the dosimetry goal is to determine the absorbed dose at some specific point in a medium under so-called *reference conditions* using a calibrated suitable detector, usually an ionization chamber. The process is known as *beam calibration* and establishes the *reference dosimetry* against which any other condition refers to, or any other detector type can be cross-calibrated. Ionization measurements require a number of corrections, coefficients, and factors to convert the detector reading into absorbed dose that depend strongly on the x-ray beam spectra. This chapter describes the beam calibration dosimetry equations, termed the *dosimetry formalism*, and the computation of the most relevant coefficients and factors.

9.1 DOSIMETRY FORMALISM

Recommendations for the dosimetry of x-ray beams, referred to as *dosimetry protocols*, have been given at the national and international level: Germany, DIN [209, 210]; Netherlands, NCS-10 [211]; UK, IPEMB [212, 213]; USA, AAPM TG-61 [214]; IAEA, TRS-277, TRS-398 and TRS-457 [67, 215, 216]. In general, protocols classify the range of kV x rays in low- and medium-energies, with generator potentials up to about 100 kV for the low-energy range and above this limit for the medium-energy range. Until recently, beam qualities have been specified in terms of the first HVL, in aluminium or copper, for the low- and medium-energy range, respectively, a criterion known to be insufficient but constrained by the availability of data.

The dosimetry formalism for kV x rays is mostly based on standards of air kerma, using an ionization chamber calibrated free-in-air in terms of this quantity. The absorbed dose to a medium, henceforth using water as standard, can be determined from either in-air or in-phantom measurements. The former is generally used for the determination of absorbed dose to water at the surface of a phantom in low- and medium-energy x-ray beams; the latter, for determining the absorbed dose at a given reference depth in a phantom using medium-energy x rays. Strictly, what is determined in both cases is *water kerma*, which for the energies involved in kV x-ray dosimetry is practically equivalent to absorbed dose to water.

For the *in-air method*, the absorbed dose to water at the surface of a water phantom in a beam of generic quality Q is given by

$$D_{w,Q}^{\text{surface}} = K_{\text{air},Q}^{\text{FIA}} \, [\mu_{\text{en}}(Q)/\rho]_{w,\text{air}}^{\text{FIA}} \, B_w(Q), \tag{9.1}$$

where

(i) $K_{\text{air},Q}^{\text{FIA}}$ is the air kerma free-in-air (FIA) at the measuring position (that is, the air kerma for the incident beam spectrum, in the absence of the phantom), obtained by multiplying the chamber reading free-in-air by the corresponding air kerma calibration coefficient $N_{K,\text{air},Q}$. The chamber reading is to be corrected for influence quantities like air pressure and temperature differences from those during the chamber calibration

(ii) $[\mu_{\text{en}}(Q)/\rho]_{w,\text{air}}^{\text{FIA}}$ is the ratio of the mean mass energy-absorption coefficients of water and air, both averaged over the photon spectrum free-in-air. It converts the air kerma free-in-air to water kerma at the same position, $K_{w,Q}^{\text{FIA}}$, that is, *water kerma free-in-air*. The μ_{en}-ratio is practically independent of field size and distance

(iii) $B_w(Q)$ is the *backscatter factor*, defined as the *ratio of water kermas* with and without the phantom present. It converts the water kerma free-in-air to the *water kerma at the phantom entrance-surface*, $K_{w,Q}^{\text{surface}}$, which is taken to be equal to the absorbed dose to water at the same position. In contrast to $[\mu_{\text{en}}(Q)/\rho]_{w,\text{air}}^{\text{FIA}}$, the backscatter factor has a strong dependence on field size and distance

This formulation has been developed under the framework of radiation therapy with kV x rays. For diagnostic and interventional radiology beams, the conceptual order of the factors in eq. (9.1) is reversed and the formulation is presented as

$$D_{w,Q}^{\text{surface}} = K_{\text{air},Q}^{\text{FIA}} \, B_{\text{air}}(Q) \, [\mu_{\text{en}}(Q)/\rho]_{w,\text{air}}^{\text{FIA+backs}}, \tag{9.2}$$

that is, the backscatter factor $B_{\text{air}}(Q)$, now defined as the *ratio of air kermas* with and without phantom scatter, converts the air kerma free-in-air to air kerma at the phantom entrance-surface, and the ratio of mass energy-absorption coefficients, now averaged over the photon spectrum free-in-air plus the backscatter contribution from the phantom $[\mu_{\text{en}}(Q)/\rho]_{w,\text{air}}^{\text{FIA+backs}}$, converts the entrance-surface air kerma to water kerma at the phantom surface.

As the two routes have to yield the same absorbed dose to water for a given beam measurement, comparing eqs. (9.1) and (9.2) yields

$$B_w(Q) \, [\mu_{en}(Q)/\rho]_{w,air}^{FIA} = B_{air}(Q) \, [\mu_{en}(Q)/\rho]_{w,air}^{FIA+backs}, \qquad (9.3)$$

which yields a harmonious link between the two different formulations [217].

For the *in-phantom method*, the absorbed dose to water at a reference depth z_{ref} is given by

$$D_{w,Q}^{z_{ref}} = K_{air,Q}^{z_{ref}} \, [\mu_{en}(Q)/\rho]_{w,air}^{z_{ref}}, \qquad (9.4)$$

where

(i) $K_{air,Q}^{z_{ref}}$ is the air kerma at the reference depth in the phantom, obtained to a first approximation multiplying the chamber reading at z_{ref} (corrected for influence quantities) by the air-kerma calibration coefficient free-in-air $N_{K,air,Q}$. The small influence on the calibration coefficient of the different spectra in air and in water can be treated as a perturbation correction factor

(ii) $[\mu_{en}(Q)/\rho]_{w,air}^{z_{ref}}$ is the ratio of the mass energy-absorption coefficients of water and air, both averaged over the photon spectrum at z_{ref}. It converts the air kerma at the reference depth in the phantom to water kerma at the same position, $K_{w,Q}^{z_{ref}}$. This ratio depends on field size and distance

Note that as the air kerma at the reference depth already includes the scatter contribution from the phantom, no backscatter factor is involved in eq. (9.4).

9.2 CALCULATION OF SPECTRUM-AVERAGED COEFFICIENTS AND FACTORS

Equations (9.1) to (9.4) show that the factors entering into the kV x rays dosimetry formalism correspond to ratios of two different quantity coefficients, kerma-related backscatter factors and mass energy-absorption coefficients for water and air. Their calculation will assume that an incident x-ray beam spectrum free-in-air, experimental or calculated, is available.

9.2.1 Backscatter factors

Backscatter factors are defined as the ratio of kermas with and without the phantom present, that is, kerma at the phantom entrance-surface to kerma free-in-air. The kermas are evaluated for water or air, for radiotherapy and diagnostic and interventional radiology beams, respectively, and the corresponding backscatter factors become defined as

$$B_w(Q) = \frac{K_{w,Q}^{surface}}{K_{w,Q}^{FIA}} \qquad B_{air}(Q) = \frac{K_{air,Q}^{surface}}{K_{air,Q}^{FIA}}, \qquad (9.5)$$

where the spectrum at the phantom entrance-surface in both surface kermas consists of the spectrum free-in-air plus the spectrum of the backscatter contribution from the phantom, "FIA + backs", see fig. 9.1. In most cases the latter requires a Monte Carlo calculation, using as input to the simulation the x-ray beam spectrum free-in-air impinging on a phantom of a given material, usually water.

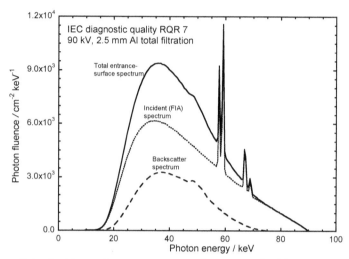

Figure 9.1: Incident photon spectrum free-in-air (FIA) for the IEC RQR 7 diagnostic radiation quality at 100 cm distance [20] and Monte Carlo-calculated backscatter spectrum for a 10 cm diameter beam at the entrance surface of a water phantom. Their sum yields the total spectrum at the phantom entrance-surface, $\Phi_k^{\text{FIA+backs}}$.

Assuming for example water kermas, and writing the explicit dependence on beam field size and distance, the backscatter factor is given by

$$B_{\text{w}}(Q, \varnothing, \text{SSD}) = \frac{\int_0^{k_{\max}} k\, \Phi_k^{\text{FIA+backs}}(\varnothing, \text{SSD})\, [\mu_{\text{en}}(k)/\rho]_{\text{w}}\, \text{d}k}{\int_0^{k_{\max}} k\, \Phi_k^{\text{FIA}}\, [\mu_{\text{en}}(k)/\rho]_{\text{w}}\, \text{d}k} \tag{9.6}$$

where Φ_k^{FIA} is the incident x-ray beam spectrum free-in-air and $\Phi_k^{\text{FIA+backs}}(\varnothing, \text{SSD})$ is the sum of Φ_k^{FIA} and the phantom backscatter component, that is, the total spectrum at the phantom entrance-surface, which in addition to the beam quality depends on the field diameter $\varnothing$ and the source-to-surface distance SSD. For the air kermas, the corresponding expression is obtained replacing "w" by "air" in the mass energy-absorption coefficients. Note that the photon spectra in the numerator and denominator remain the same in both backscatter types, as they correspond to the medium where the spectra are defined, and it is the μ_{en}/ρ-value that depends on the medium for which the kerma is determined.

Backscatter factors are usually large corrections to the water or air kerma free-in-air, particularly for large field sizes, this being the parameter for the strongest dependence of B_w or B_{air}; the variation with SSD is only a few per cent. In general, backscatter factors increase first with the beam quality and reach a maximum that depends on the incident spectrum (between 50 keV and 70 keV for mono-energetic photons), after which the values decrease [217]; the pattern is due to a complicated balance between Compton photons scattered forwards and backwards. The dependence of backscatter factors on beam quality has traditionally been associated to the first half-value layer, but a strong dependence on kilovoltage has been shown both for radiology [217] and for radiotherapy [218] x-ray beams, such that for a given HVL_1 there can be variations in the backscatter factor due to the kV of up to 10%, see fig. 9.2. The beam quality specification can thus be considered to require the pair $Q(HVL_1, kV)$.

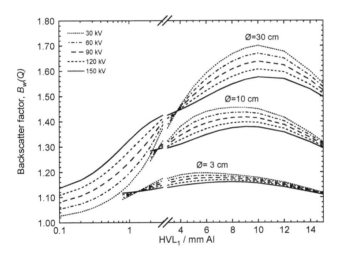

Figure 9.2: Backscatter factors $B_w(Q, \varnothing, SSD)$ for 30 kV to 150 kV incident spectra on a water phantom as a function of the HVL_1 in mm Al and for different kV and field sizes at an SSD of 100 cm. Note the log-linear break in the abscissae axis and the omission of data for beam diameters of 3 cm and 10 cm at the lowest HVLs for better visualization.

Most kV data available have been calculated for photon backscatter from water phantoms with thicknesses of 15 cm for diagnostic and interventional radiology [67, 217] and 25 cm for radiotherapy [218]. There are however situations where neither the phantom material or its thickness match a given reference configuration. X-ray measurements in liquid water can be cumbersome and, instead, phantoms made of PMMA or some kind of water-equivalent plastic are preferred in practice; however, differences in backscatter between water and other media are usually ignored. Similar constraints arise in dose determinations of small infants subject to clinical x-ray examinations, for which backscatter from small phantoms are required.

To circumvent these limitations, relevant correction factors have been formulated and data calculated to account for phantom material and thickness [219, 220]. For a phantom of arbitrary material m and thickness t, and a given field size, the backscatter factor based on, say, air kermas, is defined as

$$B_{\mathrm{air}}(Q)_{m,t} = B_{\mathrm{air}}(Q)_{\mathrm{w},15}\, f_{m,Q}\, f_{t,Q}\,, \tag{9.7}$$

where $B_{\mathrm{air}}(Q)_{\mathrm{w},15}$ is the backscatter factor for a 15 cm thick water phantom, taken as reference, and the factors $f_{m,Q}$ and $f_{t,Q}$ correct for the difference in phantom material and phantom thickness, respectively. The correction factors are given by

$$
\begin{aligned}
f_{m,Q} &= \frac{B_{\mathrm{air}}(Q)_{m,15}}{B_{\mathrm{air}}(Q)_{\mathrm{w},15}} \\[4pt]
f_{t,Q} &= \frac{B_{\mathrm{air}}(Q)_{m,t}}{B_{\mathrm{air}}(Q)_{m,15}}\,,
\end{aligned}
\tag{9.8}
$$

that is, the phantom-material factor is the ratio of backscatter factors for the material m and for water, both for a phantom 15 cm thick, and the phantom-thickness factor is the ratio of backscatter factors for an arbitrary phantom thickness t and for a phantom 15 cm thick, both of the same material. As with backscatter factors, the two phantom correction factors depend on the beam quality $Q(\mathrm{HVL}_1, \mathrm{kV})$ and field size, their dependence on source-to-surface distance being practically negligible.

9.2.2 Ratios of mass energy-absorption coefficients

Depending on the beam calibration modality and application to radiotherapy or radiology, the dosimetry formalism in eqs. (9.1) to (9.4) includes three different types of ratios of mean mass energy-absorption coefficients water-to-air. In all cases, the beam quality has a dependence $Q(\mathrm{HVL}_1, \mathrm{kV})$.

Recalling the definition of energy-fluence-weighted mean coefficient given in eq. (4.22), the water-to-air μ_{en}-ratios are calculated according to

$$
[\mu_{\mathrm{en}}(Q)/\rho]_{\mathrm{w,air}} = \frac{(\overline{\mu_{\mathrm{en}}/\rho})_{\mathrm{w}}^{\Psi}}{(\overline{\mu_{\mathrm{en}}/\rho})_{\mathrm{air}}^{\Psi}} = \frac{\displaystyle\int_0^{k_{\max}} k\, \Phi_k\, [\mu_{\mathrm{en}}(k)/\rho]_{\mathrm{w}}\, \mathrm{d}k}{\displaystyle\int_0^{k_{\max}} k\, \Phi_k\, [\mu_{\mathrm{en}}(k)/\rho]_{\mathrm{air}}\, \mathrm{d}k}\,, \tag{9.9}
$$

which depend on the type of photon spectrum Φ_k used for the averaging procedure:

(i) $[\mu_{\mathrm{en}}(Q)/\rho]_{\mathrm{w,air}}^{\mathrm{FIA}}$, for the in-air procedure in radiotherapy, is the ratio of the mean mass energy-absorption coefficients of water and air, both energy-fluence averaged over the incident photon spectrum free-in-air,

Φ_k^{FIA}. As the FIA spectrum, the ratio is assumed to be practically independent of field size and distance [218]

(ii) $[\mu_{\mathrm{en}}(Q)/\rho]_{\mathrm{w,air}}^{\mathrm{FIA+backs}}$, for the in-air procedure in radiology, where the energy-fluence average is made over the spectrum at the phantom-entrance surface, $\Phi_k^{\mathrm{FIA+backs}}$. The ratio depends on field size and distance due to the backscatter spectral component [217]. Recall that the backscatter component is usually obtained by Monte Carlo simulation

(iii) $[\mu_{\mathrm{en}}(Q)/\rho]_{\mathrm{w,air}}^{z_{\mathrm{ref}}}$, for the in-phantom procedure in radiotherapy, where the energy-fluence average is made over the photon spectrum at the depth of reference dosimetry, usually 2 cm in water, $\Phi_k^{z_{\mathrm{ref}}}$. The ratio has a dependence smaller than about 2% on field size and negligible on distance [218]. The spectrum at depth is also obtained by Monte Carlo simulation

9.2.3 Other calculation methods

The backscatter factors and water-to-air μ_{en}-ratios calculations described above have all been based upon incident spectra available experimentally or by calculation, and rely on specific Monte Carlo simulations to derive phantom backscattered or in-depth spectra. Although Monte Carlo calculations with x-ray beams are not very time consuming, the procedure might become prohibitive in terms of computer time when data for broad sets of spectra or for multiple combinations of kV, HVL, field size, and distance, need to be generated.

To overcome the constraint, it has become common [217–219, 221] to generate by Monte Carlo simulation a database of the required quantities, e.g. backscatter factors or μ_{en}-ratios, for a dense grid of monoenergetic photons with energies covering the range of realistic kV spectra. The set of simulations for calculating the various types of spectra is performed only once. An independent computer code enables the subsequent analytical calculation of the quantities for a given input spectrum by averaging the monoenergetic data over the spectrum, a calculation made in seconds. The averaging procedure is made in terms of energy-fluence for μ_{en}-ratios or of air kerma in air for backscatter factors, that is, for a kV beam of quality Q and spectrum Φ_k^{FIA}

$$B_{\mathrm{w}}(Q,\varnothing,\mathrm{SSD}) = \frac{\displaystyle\int_0^{k_{\max}} k\,\Phi_k^{\mathrm{FIA}}\,[\mu_{\mathrm{en}}(k)/\rho]_{\mathrm{air}}\,B_{\mathrm{w}}(k,\varnothing,\mathrm{SSD})\,\mathrm{d}k}{\displaystyle\int_0^{k_{\max}} k\,\Phi_k^{\mathrm{FIA}}\,[\mu_{\mathrm{en}}(k)/\rho]_{\mathrm{air}}\,\mathrm{d}k} \tag{9.10}$$

where $B_{\mathrm{w}}(k,\varnothing,\mathrm{SSD})$ are the MC-calculated values in the monoenergetic database and the air kerma in air $K_{\mathrm{air}}^{\mathrm{air}}(k)$ has been replaced by $k\,\Phi_k^{\mathrm{FIA}}\,[\mu_{\mathrm{en}}(k)/\rho]_{\mathrm{air}}$.

The averaging technique for calculating analytically data for a given spectrum, based on a Monte Carlo-generated monoenergetic database, is a rather robust method that has also been used in other radiation fields, such as megavoltage photons [222, 223], electron beams [224], proton beams [225, 226], etc.

A supplementary Python script to this chapter is available in the book's online software repository, at https://bitbucket.org/caxtus. It is called *BSFw.py* and uses the SpekPy-v2 toolkit. The script calculates $B_w(Q, \varnothing, \text{SSD})$, given a spectrum, field size and SSD. In Section 9.2.1 it was stated that SSD only weakly affects the magnitude of the backscatter factor (a few percent effect). You can verify this by calculating B_w (for a fixed spectrum and field size) for SSD values ranging from 10 to 100 cm.

CHAPTER 10

Optimizing the tube potential

I N this chapter, a simple figure-of-merit denoted the dose-normalized contrast-to-noise ratio (CNRD) is used to optimize the trade-off between image quality and radiation exposure in digital radiography. Although the approach is simplified, the predictions reflect the tube potentials used in clinical practice.

10.1 DEFINITIONS

The signal in a digital detector due to an x-ray exposure can be estimated as [108],

$$d = \mathcal{K}\mathcal{F}\mathcal{A} \int_0^{Ve} \Phi_k \left(\text{SDD}\right) \exp\left(-\sum_i^N t_i \mu_i\right) \mathcal{G}\alpha\left(k\right) k \mathrm{d}k \qquad (10.1)$$

where $\Phi_k\left(\text{SDD}\right)$ is the central-axis spectrum emitted from the x-ray tube[1] projected to the source-to-detector distance (SDD). The exponential term denotes attenuation by the subject being imaged, consisting of N tissues of different thicknesses (t_i) and linear attenuation coefficients (μ_i). The parameter $\mathcal{G}$ is the grid factor (i.e. proportion of primary radiation that passes through the anti-scatter grid), $\alpha(k)$ is the quantum efficiency (i.e. probability of interaction in the scintillator), $\mathcal{A}$ is the pixel area, $\mathcal{F}$ is the fill factor of the scintillator and $\mathcal{K}$ is the detector gain (i.e. digital values per unit energy deposited). The integration in x-ray energy, k, extends from zero up to that corresponding to the tube potential (Ve)

For our purposes, the quantum efficiency will be approximated as,

$$\alpha\left(k\right) = 1 - \exp\left(-t_\mathrm{d}\mu_\mathrm{d}\right), \qquad (10.2)$$

---

[1]This is equivalent to Φ_k^{FIA} introduced in the previous chapter, where FIA denoted free-in-air.

DOI: 10.1201/9781003058168-10

where t_d is the thickness of the scintillator and μ_d is its linear attenuation coefficient. The product $\alpha(k)k$ represents the average energy removed from the primary beam and we assume here that all this energy is deposited locally.

The variance in the detector signal may be estimated as [108, 227],

$$\sigma^2 = \mathcal{K}^2\mathcal{F}\mathcal{A} \int_0^{Ve} \Phi_k(\text{SDD}) \exp\left(-\sum_i^N t_i\mu_i\right) \mathcal{G}\alpha(k)k^2 dk, \qquad (10.3)$$

assuming there are no noise correlations between pixels (i.e. the noise is white).

We will define relative contrast between a signal or feature (d_{Sg}) and a uniform background (d_{Bg}) as,

$$C = \frac{d_{Sg} - d_{Bg}}{d_{Bg}} \qquad (10.4)$$

and the relative noise as,

$$N = \frac{\sigma_{Bg}}{d_{Bg}} \qquad (10.5)$$

The contrast-to-noise ratio is then,

$$\text{CNR} = \frac{C}{N} = \frac{d_{Sg} - d_{Bg}}{\sigma_{Bg}} \qquad (10.6)$$

We further define the dose-normalized CNR (CNRD) as,

$$\text{CNRD} = \frac{d_{Sg} - d_{Bg}}{\sigma_{Bg}\sqrt{K_{air}}}, \qquad (10.7)$$

where K_{air} is the air kerma incident on the subject being imaged[2]. The incident air kerma can be calculated as,

$$K_{air} = 1.602 \times 10^{-7} \int_0^{Ve} \Phi_k(\text{SSD}) [\mu_{en}(k)/\rho]_{air} \, k dk, \qquad (10.8)$$

where the fluence is evaluated at the source-to-skin distance (SSD) and the factor 1.602×10^{-7} converts units from keV g^{-1} to μGy.

The normalization of CNR by air kerma is convenient, as it renders the metric independent of the tube-current-time product (mAs) for the exposure.

10.2 OPTIMIZATION SCENARIOS

The figure-of-merit used for the optimization will be CNRD^2, which provides a measure of image quality achieved per unit "dose". The optimal tube potentials for different tasks will be estimated, for planar radiography with an indirect

Table 10.1: Summary of technical factors relating to the x-ray tube and detector.

Parameter	Value
Anode angle	12°
Beam filtration	3.5 mm Al + 0.1 mm Cu
Scintillator composition	CsI
Scintillator thickness	0.3 mm
Fill factor, $\mathcal{F}$	0.85
Pixel area, $\mathcal{A}$	0.1×0.1 mm^2
Grid factor, $\mathcal{G}$	0.50

digital detector based on a CsI scintillator. The technical factors relating to the beam quality and detector are summarized in table 10.1.

The imaging tasks will correspond to two types: distinguishing kidney (1 cm) from adipose tissue (1 cm) and distinguishing a solid nodule (1 cm) from lung tissue (1 cm). For both task types, calculations are performed for patient thicknesses of 15, 20, and 25 cm. The task scenarios are summarized in table 10.2. The materials and thicknesses presented are those entered into the exponential terms of eqs. (10.1) and (10.3). The SDD is assumed to be 100 cm for the first task and 180 cm for the second, with no air gap between patient and detector and an anti-scatter grid present over the detector in both scenarios.

The tungsten anode x-ray tube spectra and associated tube outputs (μGy/mAs) were estimated using SpekPy-v2 (kqp). The physics model selection of "kqp" indicates that the full spectrum model described in Chapter 6 was used.

10.3 PREDICTIONS

The contrast (C), noise (N), and incident air kerma (K_{air}) for the kidney *versus* adipose task are presented in figs. 10.1a-c, respectively. The results are provided for a tube-current-time product of 1 mAs. The relative contrast goes down slightly as the tube potential is increased, due to the reduced contribution of the photoelectric effect to the attenuation (adipose has a somewhat lower effective atomic number than kidney, amplifying contrast at lower x-ray energies). The thickness of the patient would have no effect on relative contrast for a mono-energetic beam, but here, for a poly-energetic spectrum, the extra thickness of the patient hardens the beam and marginally reduces contrast. The relative noise also declines with tube potential (because of reduced attenuation), but it does so more rapidly than the contrast. The noise also increases with the thickness of patient (because of the increased attenuation). The incident air kerma increases with tube potential, for a fixed

---

[2]This is equivalent to $K_{\text{air},Q}^{\text{FIA}}$ introduced in the previous chapter, where FIA denoted free-in-air and Q the beam quality.

Table 10.2: Summary of imaging tasks. Soft-tissue, adipose, kidney, bone, and lung are represented by the ICRU materials (Tissue, Soft, Four-component; Kidney; Adipose; Lung, Inflated; Bone, Cortical) [228].

Task type	Patient thickness [cm]	Background (Bg)	Signal (Sg)
Kidney *versus* adipose	15	14 cm soft-tissue 1 cm adipose	14 cm soft-tissue 1 cm kidney
	20	19 cm soft-tissue 1 cm adipose	19 cm soft-tissue 1 cm kidney
	25	24 cm soft-tissue 1 cm adipose	24 cm soft-tissue 1 cm kidney
Nodule *versus* lung	15	2 cm bone 6.5 cm soft-tissue 6.5 cm lung	2 cm bone 7.5 cm soft-tissue 5.5 cm lung
	20	2 cm bone 9 cm soft-tissue 9 cm lung	2 cm bone 10 cm soft-tissue 8 cm lung
	25	2 cm bone 11.5 cm soft-tissue 11.5 cm lung	2 cm bone 12.5 cm soft-tissue 10.5 cm lung

mAs, due to several factors, including the greater efficiency of bremsstrahlung generation. The difference in incident air kerma between patient thicknesses, however, is purely due to the SSD being reduced for a thicker patient, for a fixed SDD.

The contrast (C), noise (N), and incident air kerma (K_{air}) for the nodule *versus* lung task are presented in figs. 10.2a-c, respectively, again for a 1 mAs exposure. In this case, where the two materials have closer effective atomic numbers and the contrast is driven by the density difference, the contrast barely changes with tube potential and the thickness of the patient has negligible effect. The relative noise still falls precipitously with increasing tube potential, however. The differences in incident air kerma compared to the kidney *versus* adipose task are purely due to the greater SDD.

The figure-of-merit (CNRD^2) for the kidney *versus* adipose task is presented in fig. 10.3. The net effect of contrast, noise, and kerma results in a definite optimal value of tube potential, dependent on the thickness of the patient. The optimal potentials were determined as 59, 67, and 83 keV, for 15, 20, and 25 cm thick patients, respectively. The figure-of-merit is also reduced for thicker patients, indicating a need for a higher exposure (larger mAs) to attain a given CNR.

The figure-of-merit for the nodule *versus* lung task is presented in fig. 10.4. The net effect of contrast, noise, and kerma again results in a definite

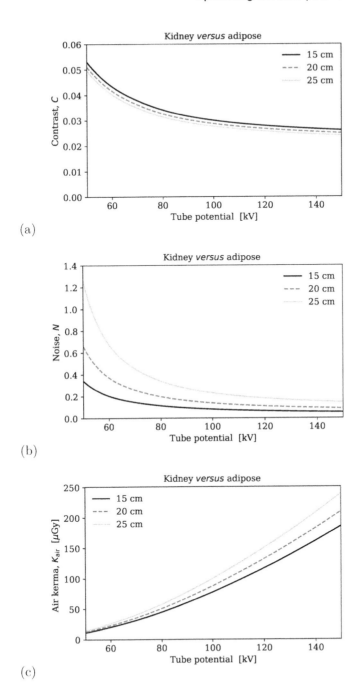

Figure 10.1: Plots of (a) relative contrast, (b) relative noise, and (c) incident air kerma against tube potential, for the kidney *versus* adipose discrimination task. Results are depicted for patient thicknesses of 15, 20, and 25 cm.

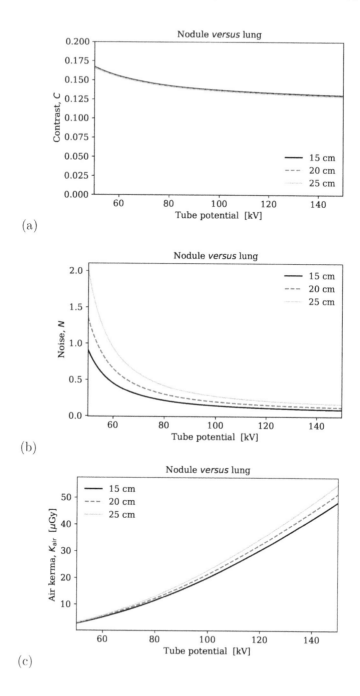

(a)

(b)

(c)

Figure 10.2: Plots of (a) relative contrast, (b) relative noise, and (c) incident air kerma against tube potential, for the nodule *versus* lung discrimination task. Results are depicted for patient thicknesses of 15, 20, and 25 cm.

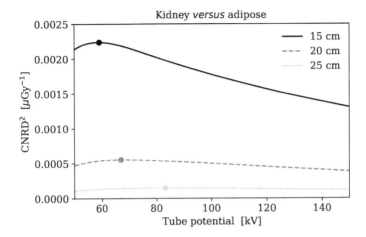

Figure 10.3: The figure-of-merit, $CNRD^2$, plotted against tube potential, for the kidney *versus* adipose discrimination task. Results are depicted for patient thicknesses of 15, 20, and 25 cm. The peak (optimal) values are indicated by solid data points.

thickness-dependent optimum for tube potential, which is substantially higher than for the kidney *versus* adipose task. The optimal potentials were found to be 116, 119, and 122 keV, for 15, 20, and 25 cm thick patients, respectively, although the figure-of-merit curve is rather flat above 100 kV. The relatively high tube potentials arise because of the presence of highly-attenuating bone.

The determinations of optimal tube potential broadly reflect clinical practice. For adults (or >20 cm), tube potentials of 70 to 80 kV are often used for abdomen radiographs (in anterior-posterior view) and tube potentials of 120 to 140 kV for chest radiographs (in anterior-posterior view). Children (or < 20 cm) are likely to be imaged with lower tube potentials.

Note that the optimal tube potential is dependent on the characteristics of the detector, as well as that of the subject being imaged. A change in the scintillator material would affect the balance between contrast and noise. Further, the results depend on the thickness of the scintillator. For example, if the thickness of the CsI was increased from 0.3 to 1.0 mm, the optimal tube potential for the kidney *versus* adipose task would increase from 67 to 87 keV, for a 20 cm patient. For the nodule *versus* lung task, it would increase from 119 to 135 keV. The absolute values of CNRD would also be higher for a thicker scintillator, as more x-rays would interact in the detector, although this advantage would have to be weighed against other factors such as a likely loss in spatial resolution.

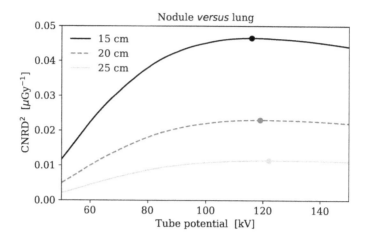

Figure 10.4: The figure-of-merit, $CNRD^2$, plotted against tube potential, for the nodule *versus* lung discrimination task. Results are depicted for patient thicknesses of 15, 20, and 25 cm. The peak (optimal) values are indicated by solid data points.

10.4   LIMITATIONS AND INTERPRETATIONS

There are several limitations to the calculations presented:

- Scatter is neglected. There will be a residual scatter contribution, even when an anti-scatter grid is present. It is possible to extend the model to include this, based on an estimated scatter-to-primary ratio [229]

- The coherent scattering contribution to the linear attenuation coefficient of the detector is included in the calculation of the quantum efficiency, $\alpha(k)$ [108]. As this contribution is not responsible for any energy transfer, strictly, it should not be included. It is however a rather small contribution to the total

- All the energy removed from the beam is assumed absorbed in the scintillator, which constitutes an *overestimation*. Even for the photoelectric effect and Compton scattering, not all the energy removed from the beam is absorbed (e.g. fluorescence escape and Compton-scattered x-rays). An alternative is to replace k with $k \times \left(\frac{\mu_{en}}{\rho} / \frac{\mu}{\rho} \right)_{d}$ in eqs. (10.1) and (10.3) [230]. However, this would be an *underestimation* of the energy absorbed, as not all fluorescence and Compton x-rays escape the scintillator

- Gain-fluctuation noise is neglected. There will be a distribution in the detected signal, for an interacting x-ray of given energy, which will contribute to the overall noise. The *Swank factor* associated with gain-fluctuation is often only slightly less than unity for detectors (i.e. little contribution to overall noise), although it can exhibit a marked drop just above a scintillator material's K-edges, due to the possibility of K-fluorescence escape [231]

- Other sources of noise such as electronic or structure noise are neglected. In many situations in digital radiography this is reasonable, as the noise is quantum limited (dominated by statistical variations in x-ray fluence and interactions) [232]

- The detector signal is assumed to depend linearly on the energy absorbed in the scintillator. This is often a reasonable assumption for detectors in radiography and even in many cases where it is not, the system can be linearized with an appropriate calibration [227]

- It is assumed that no adaptive or non-linear post-processing is applied to the images to enhance image quality (or that it can be turned off)

While extending the model to overcome these limitations would likely quantitatively affect the results, it would not be expected to change them qualitatively, with similar trends being observed.

A discussion of the nature and limitations of the figure-of-merit, is, however, warranted. The metric selected for optimization purposes was the CNR^2 divided by the incident air kerma, K_{air}. Other definitions of dose-normalized CNR are conceivable. The incident air kerma is a simple and easily calculated metric. However, while it gives an indication of the radiation the subject is exposed to, it refers to a quantity free-in-air, without the subject in-place (see the previous chapter). An improvement would be to multiply the incident air kerma with the backscatter factor, B_{air}, as the result—the entrance-surface air kerma [66]—is more closely related to patient skin dose[3]. The backscatter factor, however, depends on the beam quality and the field-size (again, see the previous chapter). Better still would be to determine absorbed doses to organs, although to do so rigorously would entail yet further loss of the approach's simplicity.

CNR itself is a commonly used metric of image quality, albeit with known limitations [233]. Not all radiological assessment tasks (and perhaps not even most) can be reduced to a decision of whether a single feature is present, against a uniform background. Regardless, CNR remains an excellent objective measure of a system's technical performance. It is therefore worth commenting on the relation of the theoretical CNR, as calculated above, to empirical estimates. When CNR is determined experimentally, it is typically performed by placing a region-of-interest (ROI) in an image, in a feature of interest and in a uniform background. The difference in the mean values between the two ROIs provides the estimate of contrast (C). The noise (N) is determined

---

[3]Note that although kerma can be considered equivalent to absorbed dose at kilovoltage energies, skin dose is specified in *tissue*, which is closely equivalent to that in *water*, but not *air*. See the previous chapter and, in particular, eq. (9.2).

from the standard deviation of pixel values in one or both of the ROIs. For detectors exhibiting white noise, the empirical CNR constructed from these estimates corresponds to that calculated above. When noise correlations are present, however, such as occur when signal is distributed across several neighbouring pixels, this is no longer true. It is in fact not meaningful to compare such empirical CNR for two systems with different noise correlations. The theoretical, uncorrelated CNR—i.e. eq. (10.6)—may be more clearly associated with the detectability of a feature in such circumstances, as it is related in a simple manner to the Rose signal-to-noise ratio (SNR) [108, 234]. The problem of empirical confirmation of the theoretical CNR remains. One solution is to rebin experimental images to larger pixels to obtain uncorrelated noise [229]. This procedure will work if the correlations are due to detector resolution (the point-spread function) or any linear post-processing filtering.

10.5 CONCLUSION

Using a spectrum model and a simple figure-of-metric representing the trade-off between image quality and dose, the optimal x-ray tube potentials were estimated for a number of tasks in radiography. The results are consistent with clinical practice.

Supplementary Python scripts to this chapter are available in the book's online software repository, at https://bitbucket.org/caxtus. The scripts are called *cnrd_kidney.py*, *cnrd_nodule.py* and *metrics.py* and use the SpekPy-v2 toolkit. Try running the script *cnrd_kidney.py* to reproduce the results of this chapter for the kidney *versus* adipose task. Now select "Gadolinium Oxysulfide" (i.e., GOS) as the scintillator instead of "Cesium Iodide" and re-run the script. How do the results change and why?

Hint: consider the K-edge energies of Cs (36.0 keV), I (33.2 keV) and Gd (50.2 keV) [167] and compare the mass attenuation coefficients of the two scintillators over the energy range.

Bibliography

[1] R. Bujila, A. Omar, and G. Poludniowski. A validation of SpekPy: A software toolkit for modelling X-ray tube spectra. *Phys. Med.*, 75:44–54, 2020.

[2] G. Poludniowski, A. Omar, R. Bujila, and P. Andreo. Spekpy v2.0: a software toolkit for modelling x-ray tube spectra. *Med. Phys.*, 48:3630–3637, 2021.

[3] W. D. Coolidge and E. E. Charlton. Roentgen-ray tubes. *Radiology*, 45:449–466, 1945.

[4] R. Behling. Chapter 2: X-ray tube physics and technology. In P. Russo, editor, *Handbook of x-ray imaging*. CRC Press, Boca Raton, FL, USA, 2017.

[5] R. Behling. Chapter 3: X-ray generators. In P. Russo, editor, *Handbook of x-ray imaging*. CRC Press, Boca Raton, FL, USA, 2017.

[6] R. Behling. Chapter 7: History of x-ray tubes. In P. Russo, editor, *Handbook of x-ray imaging*. CRC Press, Boca Raton, FL, USA, 2017.

[7] R. Behling. X-ray sources: 125 years of developments of this intriguing technology. *Phys. Med.*, 79:162–187, 2020.

[8] wikipedia:User:ChumpusRex. X ray tube in housing. https://commons.wikimedia.org/wiki/File:Xraytubeinhousing_commons.png. Accessed: 2021-10-28.

[9] IEC. *Dosimetric instruments used for non-invasive measurement of x-ray tube voltage in diagnostic radiology*. IEC International Standard 61676. International Electrotechnical Commission, Geneva, Switzerland, 2002.

[10] H. M. Kramer, H. J. Selbach, and W. J. Iles. The practical peak voltage of diagnostic x-ray generators. *Br. J. Radiol.*, 71:200–209, 1998.

[11] H. M. Kramer and H. J. Selbach. Extension of the range of definition of the practical peak voltage up to 300 kv. *Br. J. Radiol.*, 81:693–698, 2008.

[12] K. Cranley, B. J. Gilmore, G. W. A. Fogarty, and L. Deponds. *Catalogue of diagnostic x-ray spectra and other data.* IPEM Report 78. The Institute of Physics and Engineering in Medicine, York, UK, 1997.

[13] H. W. Koch and J. W. Motz. Bremsstrahlung cross-section formulas and related data. *Rev. Mod. Phys.*, 31:920–955, 1959.

[14] O. Goetze. Verfahren und glühkathoden röntgenröhre zur erzeugung scharfer röntgenbilder (line focus), 1918. Patent: DP 370 022 vom 02.

[15] J. T. Bushberg, J. A. Seibert, E. M. Leidholdt, and J. M. Boone. *The Essential Physics of Medical Imaging*, chapter 6 – X-ray production, x-ray tubes, x-ray generators. Wolters Kluwer Health, Philadelphia, PA, USA, 2011.

[16] J. T. Bushberg, J. A. Seibert, E. M. Leidholdt, and J. M. Boone. *The Essential Physics of Medical Imaging*, chapter 8 – Mammography. Wolters Kluwer Health, Philadelphia, PA, USA, 2011.

[17] J. T. Bushberg, J. A. Seibert, E. M. Leidholdt, and J. M. Boone. *The Essential Physics of Medical Imaging*, chapter 10 – Computed Tomography. Wolters Kluwer Health, Philadelphia, PA, USA, 2011.

[18] F. Verhaegen, A. E. Nahum, S. Van de Putte, and Y. Namito. Monte Carlo modelling of radiotherapy kV x-ray units. *Phys. Med. Biol.*, 44:1767–1789, 1999.

[19] C. D. Johnstone, R. LaFontaine, Y. Poirier, and M. Tambasco. Modeling a superficial radiotherapy x-ray source for relative dose calculations. *J. Appl. Clin. Med. Phys.*, 16:118–130, 2015.

[20] U. Ankerhold. *Catalogue of X-ray spectra and their characteristic data - ISO and DIN radiation qualities, therapy and diagnostic radiation qualities, unfiltered X-ray spectra.* PTB Report Dos-34. Physikalisch-Technische Bundesanstalt, Braunschweig, 2000.

[21] P. Lamperti and M. O'brien. *Calibration of X-Ray and Gamma-Ray Measuring Instruments.* Report Number 250-58. National Institute of Standards and Technology, Gaithersburg, MD, USA, 2001.

[22] Varex Imaging. Industrial x-ray tubes. https://www.vareximaging.com/products/security-industrial/industrial-x-ray-tubes. Accessed: 2021-06-04.

[23] Canon Electron Tubes & Devices. Industrial x-ray tubes. https://etd.canon/en/product/category/xray/industry.html. Accessed: 2021-06-04.

[24] X-RAY WorX. Microfocus Computed Tomography (Microfocus CT). https://www.x-ray-worx.com/index.php/en/applications-for-microfocus-x-ray-tubes/microfocus-computed-tomography. Accessed: 2021-06-04.

[25] Yxlon. X-ray and CT inspection systems. https://www.yxlon.com/en/products/x-ray-and-ct-inspection-systems. Accessed: 2021-06-04.

[26] Excillum. Metaljet x-ray sources. https://www.excillum.com/products/metaljet. Accessed: 2021-06-04.

[27] B. W. Soole. A method of x-ray attenuation analysis for approximating the intensity distribution at its point of origin of bremsstrahlung excited in a thick target by incident electrons of constant medium energy. *Phys. Med. Biol.*, 21:369–389, 1976.

[28] R. Birch and M. Marshall. Computation of bremsstrahlung x-ray spectra and comparison with spectra measured with a Ge(Li) detector. *Phys. Med. Biol.*, 24:505–517, 1979.

[29] D. M. Tucker, G. T. Barnes, and D. P. Chakraborty. Semiempirical model for generating tungsten target x-ray spectra. *Med. Phys.*, 18:211–218, 1991.

[30] M. M. Blough, R. G. Waggener, W. H. Payne, and J. A. Terry. Calculated mammographic spectra confirmed with attenuation curves for molybdenum, rhodium, and tungsten targets. *Med. Phys.*, 25:1605–1612, 1998.

[31] E. S. M. Ali and Rogers D. W. O. Quantifying the effect of off-focal radiation on the output of kilovoltage x-ray systems. *Med. Phys.*, 35:4149–4160, 2008.

[32] E. S. M. Ali and D. W. O. Rogers. Benchmarking EGSnrc in the kilovoltage energy range against experimental measurements of charged particle backscatter coefficients. *Phys. Med. Biol.*, 53:1527–1543, 2008.

[33] D. W. O. Rogers, B. Walters, and I. Kawrakow. *BEAMnrc Users Manual*. NRCC Report PIRS-0509(A)revL. National Research Council of Canada, Ottawa, 2021.

[34] I. Kawrakow, E. Mainegra-Hing, D. W. O. Rogers, F. Tessier, and B. R. B. Walters. *The EGSnrc Code System: Monte Carlo Simulation of Electron and Photon Transport*. NRCC Report PIRS-701. National Research Council Canada, Ottawa, 2021.

[35] F. Salvat. *PENELOPE-2018: A Code System for Monte Carlo Simulation of Electron and Photon Transport*. Report NEA/MBDAV/R(2019)1. OECD Nuclear Energy Agency, Boulogne-Billancourt, France, 2019.

[36] J. R. M. Vaughan. Electron flow in the conventional x-ray tube. *IEEE Trans. Electron Devices*, 32:654–657, 1985.

[37] N. A. Dyson. *X-rays in Atomic and Nuclear Physics*, chapter 2 – The continuous x-ray spectrum. Longman Group Limited, London, UK, 1973.

[38] R. W. Kuckuck. *Linear polarization of low-energy bremsstrahlung*. PhD thesis, University of California (USA), 1972.

[39] L. Kissel, C. A. Quarles, and R. H. Pratt. Shape functions for atomic-field bremsstrahlung from electrons of kinetic energy 1-500 keV on selected neutral atoms $1 \leq Z \leq 92$. *At. Data Nucl. Data Tables*, 28:381–460, 1983.

[40] S. M. Seltzer and M. J. Berger. Bremsstrahlung spectra from electron interactions with screened atomic nuclei and orbital electrons. *Nucl. Instrum. Methods Phys. Res. B*, 12:95–134, 1985.

[41] R. H. Pratt, C. D. Shaffer, N. B. Avdonina, X. M. Tong, and Viorica Florescu. New developments in the theory of bremsstrahlung. *Nucl. Instrum. Methods Phys. Res. B*, 99:156–159, 1995.

[42] E. Haug and W. Nakel. *The elementary process of bremsstrahlung*. World Scientific, Singapore, 2004.

[43] S. M. Seltzer and M. J. Berger. Bremsstrahlung energy spectra from electrons with kinetic energy 1 keV-10 GeV incident on screened nuclei and orbital electrons of neutral atoms with $Z = 1$-100. *At. Data Nucl. Data Tables*, 35:345–418, 1986.

[44] S. M. Seltzer, J. M. Fernández-Varea, P. Andreo, P. M. Bergstrom, D. T. Burns, I. Krajcar-Bronic, C. K. Ross, and F. Salvat. *Key Data for Ionizing Radiation Dosimetry: Measurement Standards and Applications*. ICRU Report 90. International Commission on Radiation Units and Measurements, Bethesda, MD, 2016.

[45] R. H. Pratt, H. K. Tseng, C. M. Lee, L. Kissel, C. MacCallum, and M. Riley. Bremsstrahlung energy spectra from electrons of kinetic energy $1 \text{ keV} \leq T_1 \leq 2000 \text{ keV}$ incident on neutral atoms $2 \leq Z \leq 92$. *At. Data Nucl. Data Tables*, 20:175–209, 1977.

[46] H. Bethe and W. Heitler. On the stopping of fast particles and on the creation of positive electrons. *Proc. R. Soc. London A.*, 146:83–112, 1934.

[47] E. Haug. Bremsstrahlung and pair production in the field of free electrons. *Z. Naturforsch.*, 30a:1099–1113, 1975.

[48] J. A. Wheeler and W. E. Lamb. Influence of atomic electrons on radiation and pair production. *Phys. Rev.*, 55:858–862, 1939. Erratum in 101(1956) 1836.

[49] M. S. Maxon and E. G. Corman. Electron-electron bremsstrahlung from a quantum plasma ($Z = 1$). *Phys. Rev.*, 163:156–162, 1967.

[50] F. Tessier and I. Kawrakow. Calculation of the electron-electron bremsstrahlung cross-section in the field of atomic electrons. *Nucl. Instrum. Methods Phys. Res. B*, 266:625–634, 2008.

[51] A. Omar, P. Andreo, and G. Poludniowski. Performance of different theories for the angular distribution of bremsstrahlung produced by keV electrons incident upon a target. *Radiat. Phys. Chem.*, 148:73–85, 2018.

[52] E. Acosta, X. Llovet, and F. Salvat. Monte Carlo simulation of bremsstrahlung emission by electrons. *Appl. Phys. Lett.*, 80:3228–3230, 2002.

[53] A. Poškus. BREMS: A program for calculating spectra and angular distributions of bremsstrahlung at electron energies less than 3 MeV. *Comput. Phys. Commun.*, 232:237–255, 2018.

[54] F. Sauter. über die bremsstrahlung schneller elektronen. *Ann. Phys.*, 412:404–412, 1934.

[55] L. I. Schiff. Energy-angle distribution of thin target bremsstrahlung. *Phys. Rev.*, 83:252–253, 1951.

[56] A. F. Bielajew, R. Mohan, and C. S. Chi. *Improved bremsstrahlung photon angular sampling in the EGS4 code system*. NRCC Report PIRS-0203. National Research Council of Canada, Ottawa, 1989.

[57] G. G. Poludniowski. Calculation of x-ray spectra emerging from an x-ray tube. Part II. X-ray production and filtration in x-ray targets. *Med. Phys.*, 34:2175–2186, 2007.

[58] G. Hernandez and F. Fernandez. A model of tungsten anode x-ray spectra. *Med. Phys.*, 43:4655–4664, 2016.

[59] A. Omar, P. Andreo, and G. Poludniowski. A model for the energy and angular distribution of x rays emitted from an x-ray tube. Part I. Bremsstrahlung production. *Med. Phys.*, 47:4763–4774, 2020.

[60] A. Omar, P. Andreo, and G. Poludniowski. *Monte Carlo-calculated depth distributions of K and L x-ray fluorescence generated by keV electrons incident upon thick targets made of Au, W, Rh, Mo, Cu, and Cr*. Mendeley Data, 2018. https://data.mendeley.com/datasets/mnr2zx92h3.

[61] X. Llovet, C. J. Powell, F. Salvat, and A. Jablonski. Cross sections for inner-shell ionization by electron impact. *J. Phys. Chem. Ref. Data*, 43:013102, 2014.

[62] D. H. Zhang, C. Z. Dong, and Z. W. Wu. Angular distribution and polarization of characteristic x-ray lines following innershell photoionization of tungsten by linearly polarized light. *J. Quant. Spectrosc. Radiat.*, 244:106844, 2020.

[63] D. E. Cullen. *EPICS2017 - Electron Photon Interaction Cross Sections*. Report IAEA-NDS-218. International Atomic Energy Agency, Vienna, AUT, 2017. Available online www-nds.iaea.org/epics/.

[64] S. M. Seltzer, D. T. Bartlett, D. T. Burns, G. Dietze, H. G. Menzel, H. G. Paretzke, and A. Wambersie. *Fundamental Quantities and Units for Ionizing Radiation*. ICRU Report 85a. International Commission on Radiation Units and Measurements, Bethesda, MD, 2011.

[65] P. Andreo, D. T. Burns, A. E. Nahum, J. Seuntjens, and F. H. Attix. *Fundamentals of Ionizing Radiation Dosimetry*. Wiley-VCH, Weinheim, Germany, 2017.

[66] J. Zoetelief, D. R. Dance, G. Drexler, H. Järvinen, and M. Rosenstein. *Patient Dosimetry for X Rays Used in Medical Imaging*. ICRU Report 74. International Commission on Radiation Units and Measurements, Bethesda, MD, 2005.

[67] G. Alm-Carlsson, D. R. Dance, L. DeWerd, H.-M. Kramer, K.-H. Ng, F. Pernicka, and P. Ortiz-Lopez. *Dosimetry in Diagnostic Radiology: An International Code of Practice*. IAEA Technical Reports Series no. 457. International Atomic Energy Agency, Vienna, 2007.

[68] A. Allisy, A. Somerwil, R. S. Caswell, K. K. Aglintsev, G. H. Aston, E. J. Axton, C. B. Braestrup, M. Chiozzotto, G. Von Droste, C. Garrett, W. Hübner, K. E. Larsson, J. S. Laughlin, K. Lidén, F. Netter, Z. Referowski, and R. Thoraeus. *Physical Aspects of Irradiation*. ICRU Report 10b. International Commission on Radiation Units and Measurements, Bethesda, MD, 1962.

[69] ISO. *X and Gamma Reference Radiation for Calibrating Dosemeters and Doserate Meters and for Determining Their Response as a Function of Photon Energy - Part 1: Radiation Characteristics and Production Methods*. ISO International Standard 4037-1. International Organization for Standardization, Geneva, Switzerland, 1st edition, 1996.

[70] L. Büermann. *PTB - Radiation qualities used for studies in radiation protection*. [WG 6.25 2010 03 09]. Physikalisch-Technische Bundesanstalt, Braunschweig, Germany, 2010. Available online http://www.ptb.de/en/org/6/.

[71] SpekPy. Welcome to the spekpy homepage. https://bitbucket.org/spekpy/spekpy_release. Accessed: 2021-08-016.

[72] J. J. Thomson. Carriers of negative electricity. Nobel Prize Lecture, December 11th, 1906. https://www.nobelprize.org/prizes/physics/1906/thomson/lecture/. Accessed: 2021-06-04.

[73] R. Whiddington. The transmission of cathode rays through matter calculations. *Proc. R. Soc. London, Ser. A*, 86:360–370, 1912.

[74] J. J. Thomson. *Conduction of electricity through gases, 2nd ed*, chapter 12 – Rays from radioactive substances. Report Number 250-58. Cambridge University Press, London, UK, 1906.

[75] N. Bohr. On the theory of the decrease of velocity of moving electrified particles on passing through matter. *Philos. Mag.*, 25:10–31, 1913.

[76] N. Bohr. On the constitution of atoms and molecules. *Philos. Mag.*, 26:1–25, 1913.

[77] A. Einstein. On a heuristic point of view concerning the production and transformation of light. *Ann. Phys.*, 17:132–148, 1905.

[78] C. G. Barkla. Polarised röntgen radiation. *Phil. Trans. Roy. Soc.*, 204:467–479, 1905.

[79] C. G. Barkla. Secondary röntgen radiation. *Nature*, 71:440, 1905.

[80] C. G. Barkla. Characteristic röntgen radiation. Nobel Prize Lecture, June 3rd, 1920. https://www.nobelprize.org/prizes/physics/1917/barkla/lecture/. Accessed: 2021-06-04.

[81] D. L. Webster. Problems of x-ray emission. *Bull. Natl. Res. Counc.*, 1:427–455, 1920.

[82] W. Duane and F. L. Hunt. On x-ray wave-lengths. *Phys Rev.*, 6:166–172, 1915.

[83] *Bulletin of the National Research Council*. National Academy of Sciences, Washington DC, USA, 1920.

[84] H. Kuhlenkampff. über das kontinuierliche röntgenspektrum. *Ann. Phys.*, 69:548–596, 1922.

[85] D. L. Webster. An approximate law of energy distribution in the general x-ray spectrum. *Proc. Natl. Acad. Sci. U.S.A.*, 5:163–166, 1919.

[86] H. Kuhlenkampff and L. Schmidt. Die energieverteilung im spektrum der röntgen-bremsstrahlung. *Ann. Phys.*, 435:494–512, 1943.

[87] H. A. Kramers. On the theory of x-ray absorption and of the continuous x-ray spectrum. *Philos. Mag.*, 46:836–871, 1923.

[88] H. Amrehn and H. Kuhlenkampff. Energieverteilung im spektrum der röntgen-bremsstrahlung dünner antikathoden in abhëngigkeit von ordnungszahl und spannung. *Z. Phys.*, 140:452–464, 1955.

[89] H. A. Bethe. Zur Theorie des Durchgangs schneller Korpuskularstrahlen durch Materie. *Ann. Phys.*, 5:325–400, 1930.

[90] H. Bethe. Bremsformel für elektronen relativistischer geschwindigkeit. *Z. Phys.*, 76:293–299, 1932.

[91] F. Bloch. Bremsvermögen von atomen mit mehreren elektronen. *Z. Phys.*, 81:363–376, 1933.

[92] F. Bloch. Zur bremsung rasch bewegter teilchen beim durchgang durch materie. *Ann. Phys.*, 408:285–320, 1933.

[93] N. A. Dyson. *X-rays in Atomic and Nuclear Physics*. Longman Group Limited, London, UK, 1973.

[94] N. Bohr. The penetration of atomic particles through matter. *Mat. Fys. Medd. Dan. Vid. Selsk.*, 18:1–144, 1948.

[95] M. J. Berger, M. Inokuti, H. H. Anderson, H. Bichsel, J. A. Dennis, D. Powers, S. M. Seltzer, and J. E. Turner. *Stopping powers for electrons and positrons*. ICRU Report 37. International Commission on Radiation Units and Measurements, Bethesda, MD, 1984.

[96] E. B. Podgorsak. *Radiation Physics for Medical Physicists, 3rd ed,* chapter 6 – Interactions of charged particles with matter. Springer, Heidelberg, 2016.

[97] A. Sommerfeld. über die beugung und bremsung der elektronen. *Ann. Phys.*, 1:257–330, 1931.

[98] G. Elwert. Verschärfte berechnung von intensität und polarisation im kontinuierlichen röntgenspektrum. *Ann. Phys.*, 426:178–208, 1939.

[99] H. K. Tseng and R. H. Pratt. Exact screened calculations of atomic-field bremsstrahlung. *Phys. Rev. A*, 3:100–115, 1971.

[100] L. Kissel, C. MacCallum, and R. H. Pratt. *Bremsstrahlung energy spectra from electrons of kinetic energy 1 keV$\leq T \leq$ 2000 keV incident on neutral atoms $1 \leq Z \leq 92$*. Report SAND 81-1337. Sandia National Laboratories, Bethesda, MD, 1981.

[101] M. J. Berger and S. M. Seltzer. Bremsstrahlung and photoneutrons from thick tungsten and tantalum targets. *Phys. Rev. C*, 2:621–631, 1970.

[102] E. Storm. Calculated bremsstrahlung spectra from thick tungsten targets. *Phys. Rev. A*, 5:2328–2338, 1972.

[103] W. J. Iles. *The computation of bremsstrahlung x-ray spectra over an energy range 15 keV to 300 keV*. NRPB Report R204. National Radiological Protection Board, Didcot, UK, 1987.

[104] D. M. Tucker, G. T. Barnes, and X. Wu. Molybdenum target x-ray spectra: A semiempirical model. *Med. Phys.*, 18:402–407, 1991.

[105] R. D. Evans. *The Atomic Nucleus*, chapter 20 – Radiative collisions of electrons with atomic nuclei. McGraw-Hill, New York, NY, USA, 1955.

[106] B. W. Soole. The effect of target absorption on the attenuation characteristics of bremsstrahlung generated at constant medium potentials. *J. Phys. B: Atom. Molec. Phys.*, 5:1583–1595, 1972.

[107] R. Birch, M. Marshall, and G. M. Ardran. *Catalogue of Spectral Data for Diagnostic X-rays*. HPA Scientific Report Series 30. Hospital Physics Association, London, UK, 1979.

[108] T. Nano and I. Cunningham. Chapter 16 – xrTk: a MATLAB toolkit for x-ray physics calculations. In J. Helmenkamp, R. Bujila, and G. Poludniowski, editors, *Diagnostic Radiology Physics with MATLAB*. CRC Press, Boca Raton, FL, USA, 2020.

[109] G. G. Poludniowski and P. M. Evans. Calculation of x-ray spectra emerging from an x-ray tube. Part I. electron penetration characteristics in x-ray targets. *Med. Phys.*, 34:2164–2174, 2007.

[110] G. Poludniowski, G. Landry, F. DeBlois, P. M. Evans, and F. Verhaegen. SpekCalc: a program to calculate photon spectra from tungsten anode x-ray tubes. *Phys. Med. Biol.*, 54:N433–N438, 2009.

[111] SpekCalc. Welcome to spekcalc. http://spekcalc.weebly.com/. Accessed: 2021-08-016.

[112] G. Hernandez and F. Fernandez. Xpecgen: A program to calculate x-ray spectra generated in tungsten anodes. *J. Open Source Softw.*, page joss.00062, 2016.

[113] A. Omar, P. Andreo, and G. Poludniowski. A model for the energy and angular distribution of x rays emitted from an x-ray tube. Part II. Validation of x-ray spectra from 20 to 300 kV. *Med. Phys.*, 47:4005–4019, 2020.

[114] A. A. Bunaciu, E. G. Udriştioiu, and H. Y. Aboul-Enein. X-ray diffraction: instrumentation and applications. *Crit. Rev. Anal. Chem.*, 45:289–299, 2015.

[115] D. L Webster, H. Clark, R. M. Yeatman, and W. W. Hansen. Intensities of K-series x-rays from thin targets. *Proc. Natl. Acad. Sci. U.S.A.*, 14:679–686, 1928.

[116] E. Storm. Emission of characteristic L and K radiation from thick tungsten targets. *J. Appl. Phys.*, 43:2790–2796, 1972.

[117] D. L. Webster, H. Clark, Yeatman R. M., and W. W. Hansen. Direct and indirect production of characteristic x-rays: Their ratio as a function of cathode-ray energy. *Proc. Natl. Acad. Sci. U.S.A.*, 14:679–686, 1928.

[118] D. L. Webster. K-electron ionization by direct impact of cathode rays. *Proc. Natl. Acad. Sci. U.S.A.*, 14:339–344, 1928.

[119] N. A. Dyson. *X-rays in Atomic and Nuclear Physics*, chapter 3 – Characteristic x-rays. Longman Group Limited, London, UK, 1973.

[120] A. Omar, P. Andreo, and G. Poludniowski. A model for the emission of K and L x rays from an x-ray tube. *Nucl. Instrum. Methods Phys. Res. B*, 437:36–47, 2018.

[121] A. M. Arthurs and B. L. Moiseiwitsch. The K-shell ionization of atoms by high-energy electrons. *Proc. R. Soc. A*, 247(1251):550–556, 1958.

[122] H. Kolbenstvedt. Energy transfer in the collision of electron beams. *Phys. Rev.*, 163:112–114, 1967.

[123] D. L. Webster. Direct and indirect production of characteristic x-rays. *Proc. Natl. Acad. Sci. U.S.A.*, 13:445–456, 1927.

[124] M. Green and V. E. Cosslett. The efficiency of production of characteristic x-radiation in thick targets of a pure element. *Proc. Phys. Soc.*, 78:1206–1214, 1961.

[125] A. Vignes and G. Dez. Distribution in depth of the primary x-ray emission in anticathodes of titanium and lead. *J. Phys. D Appl. Phys.*, 1:1309–1322, 1968.

[126] J. M. Boone and J. A. Seibert. An accurate method for computer-generating tungsten anode x-ray spectra from 30 to 140 kv. *Med. Phys.*, 24:1661–1670, 1997.

[127] J. M. Boone, Fewell T. R., and R. J. Jennings. Molybdenum, rhodium, and tungsten anode spectral models using interpolating polynomials with application to mammography. *Med. Phys.*, 24:1863–1874, 1997.

[128] A. M. Hernandez and J. M. Boone. Tungsten anode spectral model using interpolating cubic splines: Unfiltered x-ray spectra from 20 kV to 640 kV. *Med. Phys.*, 41:042101(15pp), 2014.

[129] A. M. Hernandez, J. A. Seibert, A. Nosratieh, and J. M. Boone. Generation and analysis of clinically relevant breast imaging x-ray spectra. *Med. Phys.*, 44:2148–2160, 2017.

[130] J. Punnoose, J. Xu, A. Sisniega, W. Zbijewski, and J. H. Siewerdsen. Spektr 3.0 – a computational tool for x-ray spectrum modeling and analysis. *Med. Phys.*, 43:4711–4717, 2016.

[131] L. Silberstein. Spectral composition of an x-ray radiation determined from its filtration curve. *Philos. Mag.*, 15:375–394, 1933.

[132] S. Tominaga. A singular-value decomposition approach to x-ray spectral estimation from attenuation data. *Nucl. Instrum. Methods Phys. Res. A*, 243:530–538, 1986.

[133] E. Y. Sidky, L. Yu, X. Pan, Y. Zou, and M. Vannier. A robust method of x-ray source spectrum estimation from transmission measurements: Demonstrated on computer simulated, scatter-free transmission data. *J. Appl. Phys.*, 97:124701(11pp), 2005.

[134] B. Armbruster, R. J. Hamilton, and A. K. Kuehl. Spectrum reconstruction from dose measurements as a linear inverse problem. *Phys. Med. Biol.*, 49:5087–5099, 2004.

[135] C. Leinweber, J. Maier, and M. Kachelriess. X-ray spectrum estimation for accurate attenuation simulation. *Med. Phys.*, 44:6183–6194, 2017.

[136] M. J. Flynn. WinRadImg. http://websites.umich.edu/~ners580/ners-bioe_580/index580.html. Accessed: 2021-08-016.

[137] J. M. Boone. genspec. http://ftp.aip.org/epaps/med_phys/E-MPHYA-24-1661/. Accessed: 2021-08-016.

[138] J. M. Boone. mamspec. http://ftp.aip.org/epaps/med_phys/E-MPHYA-24-1863/. Accessed: 2021-08-016.

[139] M. Bhat, J. Pattison, G. Bibbo, and M. Caon. Diagnostic x-ray spectra: a comparison of spectra generated by different computational methods with a measured spectrum. *Med. Phys.*, 25:114–120, 1998.

[140] M. Bhat, J. Pattison, G. Bibbo, and M. Caon. Off-axis x-ray spectra: a comparison of Monte Carlo simulated and computed x-ray spectra with measured spectra. *Med. Phys.*, 26:303–309, 1999.

[141] T. R. Fewell, R. E. Shuping, and K. R. Hawkins Jr. *Handbook of computed tomography x-ray spectra*. Bureau of Radiological Health, U.S. Department of Health and Human Services (FDA), Rockville, MD, USA, 1981.

[142] A. Omar. *Radiation Dose and X-Ray Beam Modelling in Diagnostic and Interventional Radiology Using Monte Carlo Methods.* PhD thesis, Karolinska Institutet (Sweden), 2020.

[143] A. Omar, P. Andreo, and G. Poludniowski. *MATLAB implementation of an analytical model for the emission of x rays from an x-ray tube.* Mendeley Data, 2020. https://data.mendeley.com/datasets/hjf5sctyt8.

[144] R. D. Deslattes, E. G. Kessler, P. Indelicato, L. De Billy, E. Lindroth, and J. Anton. X-ray transition energies: new approach to a comprehensive evaluation. *Rev. Mod. Phys.*, 75:35–99, 2003.

[145] IEC. *Medical diagnostic x-ray equipment–Radiation conditions for use in the dtermination of characteristics.* IEC International Standard 61267. International Electrotechnical Commission, Geneva, Switzerland, 1994.

[146] R. Eckhardt. Stan Ulam, John Von Neumann, and the Monte Carlo method. *Los Alamos Science*, 15:131–136, 1987.

[147] A. F. Bielajew. *Fundamentals of the Monte Carlo method for neutral and charged particle transport.* The University of Michigan, Ann Arbor, MI, USA, 2001. http://www-personal.umich.edu/ bielajew/MCBook/book.pdf.

[148] M. J. Berger. Monte Carlo calculation of the penetration and diffusion of fast charged particles. In B. Alder, S. Fernbach, and M. Rotenberg, editors, *Methods in Computational Physics*, volume 1, pages 135–215. Academic Press, New York, 1963.

[149] T. Warnock. Random-number generators. *Los Alamos Science*, 15:137–141, 1987.

[150] P. Andreo. Monte Carlo techniques in Medical Radiation Physics. *Phys. Med. Biol.*, 36:861–920, 1991.

[151] D. W. O. Rogers. Fifty years of Monte Carlo simulations for medical physics. *Phys. Med. Biol.*, 51:R287–R301, 2006.

[152] J. Seco and F. Verhaegen, editors. *Monte Carlo techniques in radiation therapy.* CRC press, 2013.

[153] R. L. Morin, editor. *Monte Carlo simulation in the radiological sciences.* CRC Press, 2019.

[154] B. van der Heyden, G. P. Fonseca, M. Podesta, I. Messner, N. Reisz, A. Vaniqui, H. Deutschmann, P. Steininger, and F. Verhaegen. Modelling of the focal spot intensity distribution and the off-focal spot radiation in kilovoltage X-ray tubes for imaging. *Phys. Med. Biol.*, 65:025002(10pp), 2019.

[155] P. V. Granton and F. Verhaegen. On the use of an analytic source model for dose calculations in precision image-guided small animal radiotherapy. *Phys. Med. Biol.*, 58:3377–3395, 2013.

[156] R. Kakonyi, M. Erdelyi, and G. Szabo. Monte Carlo simulation of the effects of anode surface roughness on x-ray spectra. *Med. Phys.*, 37:5737–5745, 2010.

[157] G. McVey and H. Weatherburn. A study of scatter in diagnostic x-ray rooms. *Br. J. Radiol.*, 77:28–38, 2004.

[158] M. R. Ay, M. Shahriari, S. Sarkar, M. Adib, and H. Zaidi. Monte Carlo simulation of x-ray spectra in diagnostic radiology and mammography using MCNP4C. *Phys. Med. Biol.*, 49:4897–4917, 2004.

[159] M. Bazalova and F. Verhaegen. Monte Carlo simulation of a computed tomography x-ray tube. *Phys. Med. Biol.*, 52:5945–5955, 2007.

[160] M. Ljungberg. The SIMIND Monte Carlo Code. In M. Ljungberg, S. E. Strand, and M. A. King, editors, *Monte Carlo Calculation in Nuclear Medicine: Applications in Diagnostic Imaging*. Taylor & Francis, Boca Raton, FL, USA, 2012.

[161] Bielajew A. F. Sempau J., Wilderman S. J. DPM, a fast, accurate Monte Carlo code optimized for photon and electron radiotherapy treatment planning dose calculations. *Phys. Med. Biol.*, 45(8):2263–91, 2000.

[162] F. Salvat and J. M. Fernández-Varea. Overview of physical interaction models for photon and electron transport used in Monte Carlo codes. *Metrologia*, 46:S112–S138, 2009.

[163] I. Kawrakow, D. W. O. Rogers, E. Mainegra-Hing, F. Tessier, R. W. Townson, and B. R. B. Walters. EGSnrc toolkit for Monte Carlo simulation of ionizing radiation transport. doi:10.4224/40001303, 2000.

[164] A. Ferrari, P. R. Sala, A. Fass, and J. Ranft. FLUKA: a multi-particle transport code. Report CERN-2005-10, European Organization for Nuclear Research (CERN), Geneva, CHE, 2005.

[165] S. Agostinelli, J. Allison, K. Amako, J. Apostolakis, H. Araujo, P. Arce, M. Asai, D. Axen, S. Banerjee, G. Barrand, et al. Geant4—a simulation toolkit. *Nucl. Instrum. Methods Phys. Res. A*, 506:250–303, 2003.

[166] T. Goorley, M. James, T. Booth, F. Brown, J. Bull, L. J. Cox, J. Durkee, J. Elson, M. Fensin, R. A. Forster, J. Hendricks, et al. Initial MCNP6 release overview. *Nucl. Technol.*, 180:298–315, 2012.

[167] M. J. Berger and J. H. Hubbell. *XCOM: Photon Cross Sections on a Personal Computer*. Report NBSIR 87-3597. National Bureau of

Standards (now NIST), Gaithersburg, MD, 1987. Available online https://www.nist.gov/pml/xcom-photon-cross-sections-database.

[168] D. Bote and F. Salvat. Calculations of inner-shell ionization by electron impact with the distorted-wave and plane-wave Born approximations. *Phys. Rev. A*, 77:04271(24pp), 2008.

[169] W. R. Nelson, H. Hirayama, and D. W. O. Rogers. *The EGS4 Code System*. Report SLAC 265. Stanford Linear Accelerator Center, Standford, CA, 1985.

[170] D. W. O. Rogers, B. A. Faddegon, G. X. Ding, C.-M. Ma, J. We, and T. R. Mackie. BEAM: a Monte Carlo code to simulate radiotherapy treatment units. *Med. Phys.*, 22:503–524, 1995.

[171] I. Kawrakow and A. F. Bielajew. On the condensed history technique for electron transport. *Nucl. Instrum. Methods Phys. Res. B*, 142:253–280, 1998.

[172] I. Kawrakow. Accurate condensed history Monte Carlo simulation of electron transport. I. EGSnrc, the new EGS4 version. *Med. Phys.*, 27:485–498, 2000.

[173] E. Storm and H. I. Israel. Photon cross sections from 1 keV to 100 MeV for elements $Z = 1$ to $Z = 100$. *Nucl. Data Tables*, A7:565–681, 1970.

[174] L. Sabbatucci and F. Salvat. Theory and calculation of the atomic photoeffect. *Radiat. Phys. Chem.*, 121:122–140, 2016.

[175] P. G. F. Watson and J. Seuntjens. Effect of explicit M and N-shell atomic transitions on a low-energy x-ray source. *Med. Phys.*, 43:1760–1763, 2016.

[176] E. S. Ali and D. W. Rogers. Efficiency improvements of x-ray simulations in EGSnrc user-codes using bremsstrahlung cross-section enhancement (BCSE). *Med. Phys.*, 34:2143–2154, 2007.

[177] V. Vlachoudis. FLAIR: a powerful but user friendly graphical interface for FLUKA. In *Proc. Int. Conf. on Mathematics, Computational Methods & Reactor Physics (M&C 2009), Saratoga Springs, New York*, volume 176, 2009.

[178] A. Ferrari, P. R. Sala, R. Guaraldi, and F. Padoani. An improved multiple scattering model for charged particle transport. *Nucl. Instrum. Methods Phys. Res. B*, 71:412–426, 1992.

[179] P. Arce, D. Bolst, M-C. Bordage, J. M. C. Brown, P. Cirrone, M. A. Cortés-Giraldo, D. Cutajar, G. Cuttone, L. Desorgher, P. Dondero, et al. Report on G4-Med, a Geant4 benchmarking system for medical physics

applications developed by the Geant4 Medical Simulation Benchmarking Group. *Med. Phys.*, 48:19–56, 2021.

[180] O. Kadri, V. Ivanchenko, F. Gharbi, and A. Trabelsi. Incorporation of the Goudsmit–Saunderson electron transport theory in the Geant4 Monte Carlo code. *Nucl. Instrum. Methods Phys. Res. B*, 267:3624–3632, 2009.

[181] S. Goudsmit and J. L. Saunderson. Multiple scattering of electrons. *Phys. Rev.*, 57:24–29, 1940.

[182] H. W. Lewis. Multiple scattering in an infinite medium. *Phys. Rev.*, 78:526–529, 1950.

[183] F. Salvat, A. Jablonski, and C. J. Powell. ELSEPA-Dirac partial-wave calculation of elastic scattering of electrons and positrons by atoms, positive ions and molecules. *Comput. Phys. Commun.*, 165:157–190, 2005.

[184] S. Jan, D. Benoit, E. Becheva, T. Carlier, F. Cassol, P. Descourt, T. Frisson, L. Grevillot, L. Guigues, L. Maigne, et al. GATE V6: a major enhancement of the GATE simulation platform enabling modelling of CT and radiotherapy. *Phys. Med. Biol.*, 56:881–901, 2011.

[185] G. Hughes. Recent developments in low-energy electron/photon transport for MCNP6. *Progr. Nucl. Sci. Tech.*, 4:454–458, 2014.

[186] D. B. Pelowitz. *MCNPX user's manual, version 2.6.0.* LANL Report LA-CP-07-1473. Los Alamos National Laboratory, Los Alamos, NM, 2008.

[187] X-5 Monte Carlo Team. *MCNP - A General Monte Carlo N-Particle Transport Code, Version 5.* LANL Report LA-UR-03-1987. Los Alamos National Laboratory, Los Alamos, NM, 2003.

[188] B. C. Franke, R. P. Kensek, and T. W. Laub. ITS Version 5.0: The Integrated TIGER Series of coupled Electron/Photon Monte Carlo Transport Codes with CAD geometry (rev 1). Report SAND2004-5172, Sandia National Laboratories, 2005.

[189] H. G. Hughes. *Treating electron transport in MCNP.* LA-UR-96-4583. Los Alamos National Laboratory, Los Alamos, NM, 1996.

[190] L. Landau. On the energy loss of fast particles by ionization. *J. Phys. USSR*, 8:201–205, 1944.

[191] O. Blunck and S. Leisegang. Zum energieverlust schneller elektronen in dünnen schichten. *Zeitschrift für Physik*, 128:500–505, 1950.

[192] D. Dixon and H. Hughes. *Validation of MCNP6 for electron energy deposition in extended media.* LANL Report LA-UR-03-1987. Los Alamos National Laboratory, Los Alamos, NM, 2015.

[193] A. Poškus. Evaluation of computational models and cross sections used by MCNP6 for simulation of characteristic X-ray emission from thick targets bombarded by kiloelectronvolt electrons. *Nucl. Instrum. Methods Phys. Res. B*, 383:65–80, 2016.

[194] J. Almansa, F. Salvat-Pujol, G. Dáaz-Londoño, A. Carnicer, A. M. Lallena, and F. Salvat. PENGEOM – A general-purpose geometry package for Monte Carlo simulation of radiation transport in material systems defined by quadric surfaces. *Comput. Phys. Commun.*, 199:102–113, 2016.

[195] J. Sempau, A. Badal, and L. Brualla. A PENELOPE-based system for the automated Monte Carlo simulation of clinacs and voxelized geometries. *Med. Phys.*, 38:5887–5895, 2011.

[196] J. Sempau. *PENELOPE/penEasy User Manual.* Technical University of Catalonia, 2020.

[197] J. M. Fernández-Varea, R. Mayol, J. Baró, and F. Salvat. On the theory and simulation of multiple elastic scattering of electrons. *Nucl. Instrum. Methods Phys. Res. B*, 73:447–473, 1993.

[198] D. E. Cullen. *A survey of photon cross section data for use in EPICS2017.* International Atomic Energy Agency, IAEA-NDS-225, rev. 1, 2018.

[199] P. Andreo, D. T. Burns, and F. Salvat. On the uncertainties of photon mass energy-absorption coefficients and their ratios for radiation dosimetry. *Phys. Med. Biol.*, 57:2117–2136, 2012.

[200] C. Valdes-Cortez, I. Mansour, M. Rivard, F. Ballester, E. Mainegra-Hing, R. M. Thomson, and J. Vijande. A study of Type B uncertainties associated with the photoelectric effect in low-energy Monte Carlo simulations. *Phys. Med. Biol.*, 66:105014(1–14), 2021.

[201] J. H. Scofield. *Theoretical photoionization cross sections from 1 to 1500 keV.* Report UCRL-51326. Lawrence Livermore National Laboratory, Livermore, CA, 1973.

[202] R. H. Pratt. Atomic photoelectric effect at high energies. *Phys. Rev.*, 117:1017–1028, 1960.

[203] R. H. Pratt and H. K. Tseng. Behaviour of electron wave functions near the atomic nucleus and normalization screening theory in the atomic photoeffect. *Phys. Rev. A*, 5:1063–1072, 1973.

[204] J. H. Hubbell. Photon mass attenuation and energy-absorption coefficients from 1 keV to 20 MeV. *Int. J. Appl. Radiat. Isot.*, 33:1269–1278, 1982.

[205] C. M. O'Brien. *Calibration of x-ray radiation detectors.* Report RPD-P-03. National Institute of Standards and Technology (NIST), Gaithersburg, MD, USA, 2017. https://www.nist.gov/system/files/documents/2017/06/19/procedure03v430.pdf. Accessed: 2021-09-09.

[206] C. Kessler and D.T. Burns. *Measuring conditions and uncertainties for the comparison and calibration of national dosimetric standards at the BIPM.* BIPM Report 18-06. International Bureau of Weights and MEasures, Sévres, France, 2018.

[207] A. Villevalde, D. T. Burns, and C. Kessler. *Beam characterization for low-energy x-rays and new reference qualities at 1 m.* BIPM Report 20-03. International Bureau of Weights and MEasures, Sévres, France, 2020.

[208] ISO. *X and Gamma Reference Radiation for Calibrating Dosemeters and Doserate Meters and for Determining Their Response as a Function of Photon Energy - Part 1: Radiation Characteristics and Production Methods.* ISO International Standard 4037-1. International Organization for Standardization, Geneva, Switzerland, 2nd edition, 2019.

[209] DIN. *Clinical dosimetry: Application of x-rays with peak voltages between 10 and 100 kV in radiotherapy and soft tissue diagnostics (in German).* DIN 6809-4. Beuth Verlag, Berlin, 1988.

[210] DIN. *Clinical dosimetry-Part 5: Application of x-rays with peak voltages between 100 and 400 kV in radiotherapy (in German).* DIN 6809-5. Beuth Verlag, Berlin, 1996.

[211] T. W. M. Grimbergen, A. H. L. Aalbers, B. J. Mijnheer, J. Seuntjens, H. Thierens, J. Van Dam, F. W. Wittkämper, and J. Zoetelief. *Dosimetry of low and medium energy x-rays, a Code of Practice for use in radiotherapy and radiobiology.* Report NCS-10. Nederlandse Commissie voor Stralingsdosimetrie, Amsterdam, 1997.

[212] S. C. Klevenhagen, R. J. Aukett, R. M. Harrison, C. Moretti, A. E. Nahum, and K. E. Rosser. The IPEMB Code of Practice for the determination of absorbed dose for x-rays below 300 kV generating potential (0.035 mm Al – 4 mm Cu HVL). *Phys. Med. Biol.*, 41:2605–2625, 1996.

[213] R. J. Aukett, J. E. Burns, A. G. Greener, R. M. Harrison, C. Moretti, A. E. Nahum, and K. E. Rosser. Addendum to the IPEMB Code of Practice for the determination of absorbed dose for x-rays below 300 kV generating potential (0.035 mm Al – 4 mm Cu HVL). *Phys. Med. Biol.*, 50:2739–2748, 2005.

[214] C. M. Ma, C. W. Coffey, L. A. DeWerd, C. Liu, R. Nath, S. M. Seltzer, and J. P. Seuntjens. AAPM protocol for 40-300 kV x-ray beam dosimetry in radiotherapy and radiobiology (AAPM TG-61). *Med. Phys.*, 28:868–893, 2001.

[215] P. Andreo, J. C. Cunningham, K. Hohlfeld, and H. Svensson. *Absorbed dose determination in photon and electron beams: An International Code of Practice.* IAEA Technical Reports Series no. 277. International Atomic Energy Agency, Vienna, 1987. (2nd ed. in 1997).

[216] P. Andreo, D. T. Burns, K. Hohlfeld, M. S. Huq, T. Kanai, F. Laitano, V. G. Smyth, and S. Vynckier. *Absorbed dose determination in external beam radiotherapy: An International Code of Practice for dosimetry based on standards of absorbed dose to water.* IAEA Technical Reports Series no. 398. International Atomic Energy Agency, Vienna, 2000.

[217] H. Benmakhlouf, H. Bouchard, A. Fransson, and P. Andreo. Backscatter factors and mass energy-absorption coefficient ratios for diagnostic radiology dosimetry. *Phys. Med. Biol.*, 56:7179–7204, 2011.

[218] P. Andreo. Data for the dosimetry of low- and medium-energy kV x rays. *Phys. Med. Biol.*, 64:205019 (19pp), 2019.

[219] H. Benmakhlouf, A. Fransson, and P. Andreo. Influence of phantom thickness and material on the backscatter factors for diagnostic x-ray beam dosimetry. *Phys. Med. Biol.*, 58:247–260, 2013.

[220] A. Almén, P. Andreo, H. Benmakhlouf, C. L. Chapple, H. Delis, A. Fransson, P. Homolka, H. Järvinen, J. Le Heron, and et al. *Dosimetry in Diagnostic Radiology for Paediatric Patients.* IAEA Human Health Series no. 24. International Atomic Energy Agency, Vienna, 2013.

[221] H. M. Kramer. SPECOM: A package for the calculation of x-ray photon spectra in water and graphite, and related kerma quantities. Unpublished report, Physikalisch-Technische Bundesanstalt, Braunschweig, 1992.

[222] P. Andreo and A. E. Nahum. Stopping-power ratio for a photon spectrum as a weighted sum of the values for monoenergetic photon beams. *Phys. Med. Biol.*, 30:1055–1065, 1985.

[223] A. Ahnesjö and P. Andreo. Determination of effective bremsstrahlung spectra and electron contamination for photon dose calculations. *Phys. Med. Biol.*, 34:1451–1464, 1989.

[224] B. A. Faddegon and I. Blevis. Electron spectra derived from depth dose distributions. *Med. Phys.*, 27:514–526, 2000.

[225] Å. Carlsson, P. Andreo, and A. Brahme. Monte Carlo and analytical calculation of proton pencil beams for computerized treatment plan optimization. *Phys. Med. Biol.*, 42:1033–1053, 1997.

[226] P. Kimstrand, E. Traneus, A. Ahnesjö, E. Grusell, B. Glimelius, and N. Tilly. A beam source model for scanned proton beams. *Phys. Med. Biol.*, 52:3151–3168, 2007.

[227] I. Cunningham. Chapter 2 – Applied linear-systems theory. In J. Beutel, H. L. Kundel, and R. L. van Metter, editors, *Handbook of Medical Imaging: vol 1. Physics and Psychophysics.* SPIE Press, Bellingham, WA, USA, 2000.

[228] D. R. White, J. Booz, R. V. Griffith, J. J. Spokas, and I. J. Wilson. *Tissue substitutes in radiation dosimetry and measurement.* ICRU Report 44. International Commission on Radiation Units and Measurements, Bethesda, MD, 1989.

[229] C. S. Burton, Mayo J. R., and I. A. Cunningham. Energy subtraction angiography is comparable to digital subtraction angiography in terms of iodine Rose SNR. *Med. Phys.*, 43:5925–5933, 2016.

[230] J. M. Boone. Chapter 1 – Applied x-ray production, interaction, and detection in diagnostic imaging. In J. Beutel, H. L. Kundel, and R. L. van Metter, editors, *Handbook of Medical Imaging: vol 1. Physics and Psychophysics.* SPIE Press, Bellingham, WA, USA, 2000.

[231] J. A. Rowlands and J. Yorkston. Chapter 4 – Flat panel detectors for digital radiography. In J. Beutel, H. L. Kundel, and R. L. van Metter, editors, *Handbook of Medical Imaging: vol 1. Physics and Psychophysics.* SPIE Press, Bellingham, WA, USA, 2000.

[232] N. W. Marshall, A. Mackenzie, and I. D. Honey. Quality control measurements for digital x-ray detectors. *Phys. Med. Biol.*, 56:979–999, 2011. https://doi.org/10.1088/0031-9155/56/4/007.

[233] P. Sharp, D. C. Barber, D. G. Brown, A. E. Burgess, C. E. Metz, K. J. Myers, C. J. Taylor, R. F. Wagner, R. Brooks, C. R. Hill, D. E. Kuhl, M. A. Smith, P. Wells, and B. Worthington. *Medical imaging–the assessment of image quality.* ICRU Report 54. International Commission on Radiation Units and Measurements, Bethesda, MD, 1996.

[234] A. E. Burgess. The Rose model, revisited. *J. Opt. Soc. Am.*, A16:633–646, 1999.

Index

absorbed dose, 39
    to water, 118
air column, 16, 105
air kerma, 1, 126
    air kerma spectrum, 41
    air kerma standards, 117
    air kerma-area product, 40
    air kerma-length product, 40
    air kerma-weighted, 41
    at entrance-surface, 40, 133
    calibration coefficient, 40, 118
    CT air kerma index, 40
    free-in-air, 118, 119
    incident air kerma, 40, 133
    reference free-in-air, 40
analytical approach, 2, 49
    definition of, 14, 57
    empirical, 66
    semi-empirical, 57, 62
    semi-empirical, order of, 57
analytical models
    Birch-Marshall, 60
    Blough, 60
    Boone, 66
    Hernandez-Fernandez, 61
    Iles, 57
    Kramers-Whiddington, 53, 57, 67
    Omar, 61
    Poludniowski, 61
    Soole, 59
    Storm, 57, 59
    Tucker-Barnes, 60
    Webster relation, 62, 65
angle
    anode, 11, 13, 15, 60, 63, 68, 104
    anode, effective, 58, 63
    electron, 15, 58, 63

    off-axis, 15, 63
    out-of-plane, 15, 58, 63, 77
    take-off, 15, 58, 67, 68, 77, 82
    tilt, 15, 63, 104
attenuation coefficient, 15, 36, 53, 58, 75, 77, 82, 125, 132
Avogadro constant, 36

backscatter factor, 118, 119, 121, 133
    phantom-material correction, 122
    phantom-thickness correction, 122
beam calibration, 117
    in-air, 118
    in-phantom, 119
beam quality, 11, 13, 40, 51, 59, 60, 98, 103, 109, 117, 121–123, 127, 133
bremsstrahlung, 10, 19, 22, 37, 38, 51, 54, 56, 57, 64, 66, 67, 75, 76, 89, 91
bremsstrahlung cross section
    Bethe-Heitler, 26, 55, 59–61, 63, 91
    Coulomb correction, 26, 55–57
    DBMO, 55
    double differential, 23
    electron-electron, 26
    electron-nucleus, 25
    Elwert correction, 55, 59–61, 63
    empirical, 60, 61
    energy-weighted, 23
    Kramers, 52, 56, 67
    partial waves, 23, 25, 55
    screening correction, 26, 28, 55–57
    Seltzer-Berger (NIST), 25, 61, 63, 67, 78, 83, 91

Milton Keynes UK
Ingram Content Group UK Ltd.
UKHW040052071024
449327UK00019B/516

9 780367 524913